THE WINE O'CLOCK MYTH

THE WINE O'CLOCK MYTH

The truth you need to know about women & alcohol

Lotta Dann

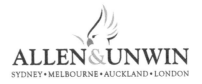

ALLEN&UNWIN
SYDNEY • MELBOURNE • AUCKLAND • LONDON

First published in 2020

Allen & Unwin
Level 2, 10 College Hill, Freemans Bay
Auckland 1011, New Zealand
Phone: (64 9) 377 3800
Email: auckland@allenandunwin.com
Web: www.allenandunwin.co.nz

83 Alexander Street
Crows Nest NSW 2065, Australia
Phone: (61 2) 8425 0100

A catalogue record for this book is available from the National Library of
New Zealand.

ISBN 978 1 98854 722 0

Cover design by Jo Pearson
Cover illustration by Kira Necheporchuk/Shutterstock.com
Text design by Megan van Staden
Set in Garamond and Caecilia
Printed and bound in Australia by Griffin Press, part of Ovato

10 9 8 7 6 5 4

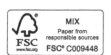

MIX
Paper from
responsible sources
FSC   FSC® C009448
www.fsc.org

The paper in this book is FSC® certified.
FSC® promotes environmentally responsible,
socially beneficial and economically viable
management of the world's forests.

For all the women

Contents

Introduction

At 3 a.m. on 6 September 2011, I woke up in my bed and immediately felt a raft of awful sensations that were not unfamiliar. My head was pounding, my mouth was dry, my stomach was churning, my bladder was bursting. I lay in the dark, feeling wretched, remembering that I'd drunk nearly two bottles of wine the night before, despite having told myself I'd have none. 'Let's have an alcohol-free night,' my husband had said as he headed off to take our two elder boys to Scouts. 'Good idea,' I'd replied, desperately trying to convince myself that yes, it was a good idea not to drink that night. It was a Monday after all, and I'd drunk a lot over the weekend. Any fool could see it made sense to take it easy.

Not this fool.

As I got out of bed and headed for the loo, I remembered that I'd raced off to buy wine while my husband and kids were out the night before, and had skulled, entirely on my own, one of the two bottles I'd bought before they got back—all while performing my normal housewifey duties. Vacuum the floor, glug, glug, glug. Close the blinds, glug, glug, glug. Get the baby into his jammies, glug, glug, glug. I was well practised at this routine, having been a high-functioning boozer for many, many years.

Shuffling in the half dark, almost at the bathroom, a memory started surfacing in my foggy brain and it stopped me in my tracks. Had I? Had I hidden the empty first bottle? The thought sharpened into focus. Holy shit—I had. I'd hidden the empty bottle to conceal the fact that I'd finished it alone, in the space of an hour. Right before they'd got back, I'd crouched down and tucked it away at the rear of the pantry, behind the spare boxes of tissues. When they walked in the door, I had the second bottle out and pretended it was the only one.

I changed course from heading for the bathroom and went instead to the kitchen to retrieve the empty bottle from its dark hiding place, gently placing it into the recycling bin so as not to wake anyone, shame flaming in my ears. Sitting on the toilet a minute later, I put my head in my hands and silently cried. This wasn't an unfamiliar position for me to be in—on the toilet at 3 a.m. feeling sick and guilty about how much I'd drunk the night before. But now I had a new dysfunctional behaviour to worry about. I'd lied. I'd lied about how much wine I'd had and I'd hidden an empty bottle. I was a person who hid empty bottles, and everyone knows that's classic alcoholic behaviour. Why the hell had I done it? Why?

I'd never lied about my intake before because, well, why should I? It was perfectly okay to be a nightly drinker. Five o'clock is wine o'clock—everyone has a drink at five o'clock. I certainly had for over twenty years. This was just how I lived, and all the messages around me, coming from friends, family, our wider society and the environment I lived in, stated very clearly that having a nightly drink was a normal, acceptable thing to do. I'd always been led to believe that drinking alcohol was the perfect way to end the day, a reward for working hard, the trigger to relax. I deserved it; I'm a hard-working mother of three, running a household, working as a freelance journalist while also studying part-time towards a masters degree. A busy, successful woman—surely a nightly wine was a decent reward for all I was achieving?

But my normal, nightly wine habit was getting out of control. I needed more and more wine to feel 'full' of an evening, and struggled to go a single day without. I made deals with myself about how much I was going to drink and constantly broke them. I was frequently sloppy, slurry, messy. There was vomiting and stumbling. My once 'normal' habit was obviously progressing to something more dangerous. I'd been acutely aware of this, and had been engaged in a dialogue with myself to try to moderate my intake. But nothing was working. And now this—hiding a bottle, a new dysfunctional behaviour at a time when I was trying to improve things. I could see where I was heading, and it wasn't good.

I sat on the toilet crying, feeling utterly stuck and miserable. And totally alone. No one around me understood my inner turmoil with regard to alcohol, even if I tried to explain it. They were wired differently, and would say things like, 'Just have one if you're worried' (as if it was that easy). So what could I do? I wanted to keep drinking, but at the same time I didn't, knowing it was a growing problem for me. It was a horrendous place to be. I felt shameful and pathetic. Normally quite an optimistic person with a kind inner voice, I had become a very negative thinker. I told myself constantly that I was weak for not being able to control my intake or change my behaviour, that I was broken. My self-esteem and self-worth were at an all-time low.

This was my personal rock bottom.

Then suddenly, through the tears, pounding temples and sick guts, I had a moment of clarity. A teeny, tiny thought popped into my head: *The problem isn't me. The problem is the alcohol.*

A little thought, but oh so powerful. It repeated itself. *The problem isn't me. The problem is the alcohol.* And then this: *If I take the alcohol away, the problem has gone.* And with these thoughts I found a small sense of strength. I managed to tap into the tiny part of me that still believed in myself, that had some power. *The problem isn't me. The problem is the alcohol. If I take the alcohol away, the problem has gone.* I seized on that tiny feeling of strength, got up off the loo, and made a monumental decision. I was going to quit booze—completely. No more trying to control and moderate. No more attempting to do deals with myself. No more. Alcohol was going from my life and I would teach myself how to be a non-drinker.

How completely and utterly terrifying. All my years I had been conditioned to believe that alcohol was a vital ingredient if you wanted to lead a full, fun life. Facing the prospect of never drinking again was like standing on the edge of a cliff, staring into a black abyss. But I knew something had to change, and this was it. Alcohol had to go. I had no idea what was to come.

Getting sober transforms every single aspect of my life. After my sad and shameful hiding-the-bottle moment, I go through a monumental turnaround. I quickly come to the realisation that for most of my adult life I've been an A-grade emotion-avoider, using alcohol to help me hide from uncomfortable feelings. Coming to terms with my sadness and anger (plus every other emotion you can name) is a painful and messy process. I slowly discover how to embrace fear and vulnerability, which enables me to properly connect not only with myself, but with all the people around me. I learn how to recognise the workings of my brain, how to distance myself from my thoughts, and how to ground myself in my body and the moment. I learn how healing tears are, and how pure joy makes my breath catch in my throat.

I also discover new, authentic ways to relax and unwind, and how to socialise without a drink (or eight) in my belly. Mingling with others while sober is awfully awkward and uncomfortable at first but, like everything else after quitting, it eventually becomes my new, comfortable normal. I realise that parties and events succeed or fail based on a range of factors that don't include the type of liquid I have in my glass.

In short, I discover that I don't need alcohol to live a full, fun life, and that all the messages I've been fed my whole life regarding alcohol are complete and utter bullshit. My whole drinking career—twenty-plus years of it—was built on a vast array of misapprehensions and misconceptions.

While all this personal growth is occurring and all these revelations are coming to me, I also experience a transformation in my professional life. Sobriety unwittingly leads me to discover my true strength, which is writing about personal stuff and what is going on inside my head. To backtrack: two days after my moment of clarity on the toilet, I decided that writing would be the main tool in turning my life around. So I decided to write myself a letter every day to keep myself focused and motivated, and allow me to stay on top of my thoughts. Because I am a fast typer I decide to put these personal letters into a free online blogging template, assuming that, given my blog would be one of millions, it would remain private and unread by others. I call my blog 'Mrs D is Going Without', and pour my heart out into it day after day. I write about what I'm doing, how I'm struggling, my trials and triumphs. I write freely with no filter, unconcerned with what anybody else thinks because no one reads my words but me. Until, that is, they do.

As the weeks pass, people start discovering my blog, reading my 'private letters', and leaving me lovely comments. It's incredible! Each comment feels like a hug—or at least a bloody good handshake. They empathise, sympathise, offer advice and share their own, similar, experiences. I discover my tribe. No longer am I going it alone—far from it. I discover that there are many, many people just like me, struggling to control alcohol, feeling miserable, stuck and alone, searching the internet for support. This is a phenomenal revelation, and helps strengthen my resolve to stay sober. As the months go on and my readership grows, an incredible community of support blossoms around my blog. It is absolute gold.

After three years of not drinking, learning how to navigate the world as a sober person and blogging my heart out, I get a very strong urge to tell my story more widely, buoyed by the feedback I'm getting online and the knowledge that there are countless others out there just like me. I suspect that, for each one of us finding online support for ditching alcohol, there must be many more who aren't. I also know there are likely to be many people who aren't yet at the point of seeking help, but are feeling stuck, miserable and alone, just like I was in the years leading up to my rock bottom. I send an email to a publishing house to see if they agree I have a story worth telling, and they email me back to say yes! So, with a signed book deal on the shelf, I proceed to write my first memoir.

I'm almost ready to submit the manuscript for *Mrs D is Going Without* when I decide I'll add a list of helpful websites at the back that readers can visit if they want more help. In the process of compiling the list I reach out to a woman who heads up a government agency that supports those who work in the addiction sector. We meet for a coffee, and it very quickly becomes apparent that there's a real lack of websites where people can join together to support one another with their drinking issues. Without having really planned on it, I blurt out an idea I've got about a community website where people can come together safely and anonymously and support one another. 'My blog is a bit limited in what it offers,' I explain, 'but I get over a thousand hits a day. Wouldn't it be great if those people could do more than just leave me a comment? Wouldn't it be great if they could talk among themselves?' She agrees, and a couple of weeks later has pulled in two other agencies to help fund and support the building of a new community recovery website.

So now I've got a new amazing website being built that is really going to help others, and a book about to come out. My publisher starts organising media interviews to help promote the book, and a high-rating news programme, TVNZ's *Sunday*, decides they want to do an extended feature on me. I nervously agree, and just keep reminding myself about the people I want to reach. To help with the nerves and feelings of vulnerability I form a vision in my mind of an imaginary woman, someone in the same position I was in three years ago, who is miserable and alone, stuck in a boozy hellhole, not able to see a way out. 'I'll do it for her,' I tell myself.

The TV crew arrives and they film intensely over four days. I cry on camera recounting the story of hiding the bottle, and when they finally depart I fall into bed, exhausted and emotionally wrung out. When the show goes to air a couple of weeks later, I watch it in my pink onesie, feeling nervous but excited. The journalist has done a good job and she tells my story without overly dramatising things or making me look like a dickhead.

The reaction is immediate. On the night my story goes to air my blog, averaging around 1500 hits a day by now, gets 45,000 hits. I am flooded with hundreds of emails and private messages, all saying a version of the same thing: 'I'm just like you.' It's incredibly moving and strengthening. I reply to each and every one, telling them about the community website we're about to launch, encouraging them to join. The book is released and the website launches. New members begin signing up to livingsober.org.nz immediately. We soon have hundreds of people on our site talking honestly and kindly to one another, working hard to reassess their relationship with alcohol. We share, empathise, advise and support one another. It's all bloody awesome.

Years go by and I rack up the milestones. Four years sober. Five. I build a reputation as a recovery advocate, my social-media accounts are busy and I get called on regularly by the media to talk about sobriety and recovery. I'm invited to speak at many public events, fundraisers and conferences (it takes me about 30 talks before I stop crying when mentioning hiding the bottle). I'm even invited to speak at Parliament. I write another memoir, *Mrs D is Going Within*, canvassing all the tools I've been working on to help me deal with life in the raw (things like mindfulness and gratitude). Living Sober goes from strength to strength: we celebrate 3000 members, then 4000, 5000. People, largely women, swarm into our safe and anonymous space, opening up about what's really going on with their drinking. For so many of them, their struggle is hidden, just as it was for me. Outwardly they're managing their lives, but under the surface things are not good at all. They're drinking more than they'd like, sleeping terribly, constantly managing hangovers, feeling guilty, strung out, out of control, miserable, conflicted and low. With the kind and non-judgemental support of others in our community, many of them begin the hard work of turning their lives around. It's heartening and enriching to watch the transformations occur. Many people succeed.

By the end of 2018 things are going great. I'm happily sober, my work life is stimulating and I'm communicating online daily with hundreds of brave and amazing people who inspire me greatly. But I'm feeling unsettled. There's a growing concern nagging away inside me, and as time goes on I'm finding it impossible to ignore. It's alcohol, of course, and the massive disconnect between what I'm hearing from people about their struggles with it, and the lie being perpetuated by how it's positioned in our society. This disconnect strikes me as utterly crazy and hugely damaging; I almost can't believe it's going on. Can't others see what I see? Alcohol is negatively affecting the lives of so many people—women especially—yet you wouldn't know it by walking around. It's almost as if their experiences aren't real, as if my experience isn't real. To the uninitiated (like, say, a child or an alien who has just landed on planet Earth) you'd think alcohol was simply a harmless, ordinary commodity. But for so many of us it's not. Where is our truth reflected?

It bothers me. It bothers me that it's allowed to be this way. It bothers me that we've created an environment that doesn't reflect all of what's going on. It bothers me that only one side of the picture is visible. It bothers me that there's a huge amount of shame and stigma for people who struggle to manage this addictive drug. It bothers me that we've created an environment where it's really difficult for people to admit their truth. It bothers me that the majority of people don't seem to know what's really going on. It bothers me that I hear from so many women who are feeling so awful. It bothers me that they're desperate to change but the environment is stacked against them. It all bothers me a great deal.

And so I decided to write this book.

This book presents the truth. It lays bare the situation we're in right now with regard to alcohol. It uncovers how normalised and glorified we've let this drug become, and unpicks the impact alcohol is having on our physical, emotional and mental health. It reveals how the liquor industry targets and manipulates women, looks at what might be causing so many of us to drink unhealthy amounts, and it discusses what can be done if you want to turn things around for yourself.

How this book works

This book is broken into five parts, each containing a broad theme exploring a different aspect of the subject of women and alcohol. Part One looks at alcohol's ubiquitous place in our society, how we use it and what we believe it does. Part Two analyses the many different ways that alcohol impacts on our bodies and minds. Part Three examines the liquor industry's sales and marketing tactics and the manipulation that goes on, particularly on social media. Part Four looks into the potential causes and reasons behind why so many of us are drinking. And Part Five explores what it's like to not drink alcohol, and how to shift drinking habits.

Each of these parts contains chapters written by me, interspersed with stories from women about their personal relationship with alcohol, told in their own words. I have included these stories to reveal the truth about women's complex relationships with alcohol, and to counteract the myths that are so often fed to us about how positive and uncomplicated our drinking habits are. The stories have been placed in the book at a point where some aspect of the woman's story relates to the topic currently being discussed, but in reality every story could have gone in five or more different places, such is the depth and richness of what each contains. Half of these stories come from women I dealt with through my work managing livingsober.org.nz. They had all previously shared their stories on that site, and when I approached them again to ask if they'd go into more detail about their drinking history for my new book they all agreed. The others I found by putting a call out on my Facebook page (Mrs D is Going Without) asking for women who were currently habitually drinking to share their stories. I was inundated with replies, choosing ten from the more than 60 women who put their hands up, offering to speak with me.

I interviewed each woman at length, over the phone or in person, recording the conversations. I then transcribed the interviews and typed up each story before emailing them back to the women. I invited them to read over their stories and let me know if they'd like any changes made for privacy, accuracy or comfort reasons. Half of the women have chosen to use a pseudonym.

The stories contained within these pages are powerful, honest, revealing and raw. They are as unremarkable as they are remarkable, because the reality is, if you talk to any women openly and honestly about her relationship with alcohol and how it's played out across her lifespan, you will likely hear a moving story containing plenty of emotion and pain.

Part One

OUR BOOZY WORLD

1.

Here, there
and everywhere

Did you know that half of the humans on this planet don't drink alcohol? Crazy but true. Around 50 per cent of the world's population never touches alcohol, ever. There are many reasons why a person might abstain from drinking, but for most of the world's non-drinkers the simple reason they stay permanently sober is that they live in countries where alcohol is banned. Either it's fully illegal, like in Afghanistan or Saudi Arabia, or it's heavily restricted or banned for religious reasons, stopping it from becoming an ingrained part of life, like in Pakistan or Egypt.

That's certainly not the case where I live. 'An ingrained part of life' is how I would describe the situation in New Zealand with regard to alcohol. I literally can't go more than a few hours without bumping into some alcohol somewhere. It is impossible to avoid (trust me, I've tried). Alcohol has infiltrated, enmeshed, embedded itself into every little nook and cranny of my environment, as it has in most other countries in the Western world. So completely has alcohol been embraced by our societies, it's become an accepted part of the landscape: we're so accustomed to seeing it everywhere that we almost *don't* see it anymore. When I first started writing this chapter I made a big effort every day to look out for alcohol—either the real, liquid stuff, or images of or references to it. Crazy as it sounds, I had to really concentrate to remind myself throughout each day to do this—I was so accustomed to seeing it everywhere that I kept missing it! But, boy, if you really open your eyes and start looking out for it like I did, you'll become all too aware just how saturated we are in booze.

Firstly, it's for sale everywhere. You can buy alcohol at restaurants, cafés, bottle shops, grocery stores, supermarkets, vineyards, breweries, hotels and taverns. It's actually pretty unusual to enter any sort of social establishment and not find booze on offer; most places where humans gather have a licence to sell booze. 'We've mapped it in Auckland, and it's pretty much in every single retail precinct,' the head of Alcohol Healthwatch, Dr Nicki Jackson, told me. 'Wherever there's a shop, there's a bottle store.' In my suburb alone, you can buy alcohol from nine different places: two large supermarkets that boast massive beer and wine sections, a smaller grocery store with a sizable beer and wine section, two dedicated liquor stores, two gastropubs and two other licensed restaurants. If I don't want to leave home I can get alcohol delivered directly to my door by any one of a number of online retailers or mail-order companies.

You can buy alcohol at the movies, at the museum, at concerts and at major sporting events. You can book a winery tour, go on a brewery trail, take part in a bar crawl or attend an alcohol-themed festival (Beervana, Winetopia and Oktoberfest are booze-based festivals held in my city each year). Often times you don't even need to intentionally be looking to buy alcohol to end up having some. I've been offered a drink at the hairdressers, inside the beauty salon, at the day spa, in a realtor's office and onboard a plane. School and charity fundraisers often offer a glass of bubbles as part of the ticket fee. Even events devoted to health and wellness often have alcohol attached. Wine meditation—it's a thing! So is beer yoga. A friend of mine recently took part in a charity race run by a large multinational company—a fundraiser for three emergency medical charities. The course was designed to finish at a winery so participants could have 'plenty of opportunity to relax'. Props to the company for raising thousands of dollars, but can't they see the irony in attaching alcohol to an event raising money for cash-strapped medical services that are kept extra-busy thanks to alcohol? (One in four admissions to hospital emergency departments is alcohol-related.)[1]

I had a woman tell me once about a conversation she'd had with a guy who was helping organise a charity walk raising awareness of mental health. He told her he was in charge of organising drinks for the event, and that he was thinking of offering beer to participants as they ended the walk. Gobsmacked, she told me she'd looked him straight in the eye and said, 'The last bloody place I want to see booze is at an event for mental health!' It's remarkable to think this guy wasn't aware of how alcohol can increase the symptoms of mental-health problems like anxiety, depression or bipolar disorder.[2]

While alcohol itself isn't literally everywhere (it wasn't available at the dentist's office where I just went for a check-up—although I did drive past six places that sell it on the way there), images of it and references to it are. The glossy magazine I read while waiting to get my teeth drilled was full of images of people drinking alcohol, as most glossy magazines usually are. Images of happy people drinking alcohol are everywhere in giant form as well, thanks to all the posters and billboards that are dotted around. Sometimes these aren't even specifically advertising alcohol! I spotted one selling homewares the other day that showed a group of women merrily clinking wine glasses, and another for a clothing brand that had gorgeous millennials in winter knits nursing amber-filled tumblers as they gathered around an open fire.

Then of course there are the many products related to or referencing drinking. Most shopping trips, virtual or in the real world, have me encountering drinking vessels, cocktail shakers, wine racks, beer holders, corkscrews, bottle openers, bar tools, coasters and decanters. Not to mention all of the 'decorative' items covered with jokey images and slogans such as: 'I cook with wine, sometimes I even add it to the food'; 'Stressed, blessed and wine obsessed'; 'Don't cry over spilled milk, it could have been wine'; and 'Step aside coffee, this is a job for wine'. I could fill an entire chapter with jokey lines about alcohol; they're on everything from T-shirts to aprons to mugs to coasters to tea towels to large wooden signs for hanging in your kitchen if you so desire. As for greeting cards, don't get me started. Every time I go to choose a birthday, anniversary or some other type of congratulatory card I end up sifting through a bunch about alcohol: 'It's your birthday, time to get wrecked!'; 'Let's get into the holiday spirits!'; 'Dear wine, be my valentine'. Sometimes it's hard to find a card that *isn't* booze-related.

Even my virtual world is saturated with alcohol. The news websites I visit daily devote entire sections to 'Food and Wine' (I just logged in to a major local news site and saw the headline: 'Wine company using smart search technology to make ordering easier'), and our public-service radio station regularly features liquor experts offering reviews and recommendations, as does our nationwide talk radio network and other smaller local stations. Many of these liquor experts have their own websites full of tasting notes and reviews, as do hundreds of other outlets and companies. There are thousands of alcohol-related websites full of articles, cocktail recipes, food matches, winemaking details, professional reviews, bar guides, city guides, games, sales, deals and promotions. I just googled 'alcohol tasting notes' and got 22 million results in less than a second. 'Alcohol recommendations' got me 221 million results just as quickly. There are also numerous apps offering tasting notes, food matches, winemaking details, professional reviews, memes, videos and gifs centred on alcohol.

Speaking of alcohol-related memes, videos and gifs, social media is groaning under the weight of them. Thousands every minute are being shared, liked and commented on, many originating from pages and accounts that have thousands—sometimes millions—of followers.

Television doesn't escape alcohol's images either—far from it. According to the website actionpoint.org.nz, a scene depicting alcohol occurs on prime-time television in New Zealand every nine minutes.[3] I've lost count of the number of times I've watched a character in a dramatic production arrive home, dump their bag, kick off their shoes and pour themselves a large glass of wine. It's very unusual to witness any group of adults socialising together on TV without most of them holding a drink in hand. The reality TV genre is particularly booze-soaked: Real Housewives are always getting drunk and messy; love-seekers on *The Bachelor* and *The Bachelorette* sup alcohol on dates; the hosts of *Location, Location, Location* are forever doing real estate deals at the pub. And let's not even get into the shows that are entirely centred on young people getting hellishly drunk together (I'm looking at you, *Geordie Shore, Floribama Shore* and *Jersey Shore: Family Vacation*).

If you truly open your eyes you'll start easily noticing how booze-saturated we are. Our physical environments are liberally splashed with alcohol, it's right throughout our media landscapes, and it's all over our virtual worlds—enmeshed, embedded and visible quite literally in every little nook and cranny. And not only is it enmeshed, embedded and visible everywhere, but it's everywhere *being portrayed as a good thing*. When travelling around my suburb, city or country, listening to the radio, watching TV, scrolling through social media or surfing online, I get little to no messaging that there is a dark or dangerous side to this product. If I dig a little deeper and make a real effort to find counterpoints to the overwhelmingly positive messages about alcohol, I *can* find them. But, to the casual observer, alcohol is only ever presented as a delightful liquid that has magical powers to make every and any occasion better, with no real downsides. No surprises then that alcohol is our favourite drug, one we drink millions of litres of annually.

2.

Veronica

*'Without a doubt the environment
contributes to my habit.'*

My dad used to drink beer, not every day but regularly. My mum hardly ever drank. She told me once she didn't like the feeling of losing control. From when I was about maybe eight to ten years old, Dad would give me the occasional shandy, and I remember quite liking that. So I guess I was having my first taste of alcohol from a relatively early age.

I was sixteen when I started properly drinking, and I remember having a few horrible experiences on cheap wine. There's a photo somewhere of me with my first hangover, spewing my guts out with my poor friend holding my hair back. I just thought, *This is what you pay for having a good time.* That first experience put me off for a wee while, but I never learned any sense of moderation. Binge drinking was normal, and I did it fairly regularly as I got older. There was a dangerous undercurrent of it being something slightly subversive, a kind of freedom somehow. There was even some kind of heroic vibe around what you could drink, how loose you could get, how much fun you could have, the naughty stuff you'd get up to.

I went straight from school to university, got a degree, then took a year off. I continued to binge drink pretty regularly through that time. I have quite a few different memories of fairly disastrous moments related to alcohol. There was one episode where it was my friend's twenty-first birthday and we went to a graveyard and had a picnic. I got really shit-faced on Jack Daniel's, or something heinous, and professed to him that I was in love with him. He was gay, so that didn't go down very well. He ended up abandoning me there, and I woke up in the middle of the night screaming, having no idea where I was. Some local people came, took me to their house and tried to get me to ring someone to pick me up, but I had a hard time remembering any phone numbers. Eventually I got a friend to come and pick me up. That was pretty disastrous.

At that time in my life I had such a shitty sense of myself. I come from some hideous family dysfunction that left me feeling pretty trapped inside myself, and I definitely have social awkwardness. I'm way less shy now, and alcohol has always helped me to loosen up, come out of my shell and actually connect with people. I'm so aware that it needn't be the only way I do it, but it's just a pattern, a habitual thing. Drinking has always simultaneously been a release from how bad I feel and also a means of digging myself further into feeling like shit.

I went back to university and did an honours year, then took on a massive masters that turned into a PhD, which ended up falling over. If I'd taken on just a part of what I was embarking on it probably would have been doable, but I just ended up abandoning it because it was too huge. After that I moved away to a very remote area for eight years and lived in the bush without electricity or a phone line. That was a great experience, but I was very isolated and never really found my community there. I'm back in the city now.

I'm aware that I'm drinking too much, too often. I've got a gorgeous group of friends and we all love drinking together. We get together at each other's houses and cook delicious food, drink wine, dance, gasbag and just have a really fucking good time. The whole getting drunk together thing is so ingrained; it's how we relate and enjoy each other's company. I fear losing that if I'm not drinking. One of my friends said to me recently that she feels like she's an alcoholic but on the mild end of the spectrum, and another one is definitely an alcoholic and isn't really facing it at all. I don't know what it would be like if I turned up and announced I was not drinking. I can imagine myself hanging back more because alcohol liberates me from my inhibitions and my weirdness around relaxing with people. So I don't know, I guess it remains to be experimented with eventually. It is a little bit of a scary prospect, though from time to time I do have an alcohol-free night—maybe once a fortnight.

Without a doubt the environment contributes to my habit. I'm in this schizophrenic awareness of being able to see so clearly on an intellectual level how booze-saturated our culture is, yet still participate in it myself. So there is a disjunction there. It's an uncomfortable place to be, but at this point I think I'm just gonna probably keep going as I'm going. I don't feel like I'm on the slippery slope; I feel like I'm in a holding pattern. I guess that's why I'm not hugely motivated to change right now.

I very regularly think to myself that I'll probably give up alcohol completely one day. But I don't feel ready to do that yet. It is a struggle imagining how to live sober and still enjoy my life and have the kind of fun I'm having at the moment. I can't imagine what the trigger will be for me to stop. There may be an interim period where I drink less, and less often. Or it might be that I simply make the decision one day. I hope it doesn't take a bloody disaster. Even though I'm aware that I'd probably be better off in lots of ways if I gave up drinking, I'm not motivated to do it, because it's okay for me right now. There is a problem; it's just not a glaring, painful, sharp-edged problem at this point.

3.

Treat, reward, celebrate, soothe

Put your hand up if you'd love to live in a world where alcohol wasn't so normalised and glorified. My hand's up. I don't think it needs to be outlawed completely—that's not necessary, or fair on those who have a casual relationship with the stuff—but I do wish we could pull back a bit from the unmitigated devotion our society seems to have to it. I'd love it if alcohol wasn't front and centre all the time, given the power to make every event and gathering seem worth attending. I know there are many others who feel like I do, but it would appear we're in the minority. Most people seem to firmly believe that alcohol is a vital ingredient of every occasion. They must do, or our world wouldn't be so booze-soaked.

I'm not judging. I totally get it. I was fully of that mindset for most of my life, believing unquestionably that alcohol was an essential ingredient for a full and fun life. It's no surprise that I felt this way given we've been sold this idea our entire lives. It's almost impossible not to soak up the pro-drinking messages as we move around our environment. What says alcohol is good for you more than endless images of healthy people drinking it? What says alcohol is harmless more than booze sitting alongside bread and milk in the supermarket? What says alcohol solves your problems and eases your mind more than countless slogans claiming exactly that all over products and greeting cards? What says alcohol is an intellectual pursuit more than countless experts pontificating on the subject of booze?

From infancy through to adulthood, we're bombarded with messages—both overt and subliminal—that reinforce the idea that alcohol is a positive and harmless thing, and that drinking it is the best way to treat and reward ourselves, celebrate and have fun with others, and relax and ease our troubled minds. As Allen Carr, author of *The Easy Way to Stop Drinking: A revolutionary new approach to escaping from the alcohol trap*, puts it: 'From the moment we are born, our young brains are bombarded daily with information telling us that alcohol quenches our thirst, tastes good, makes us happy, steadies our nerves, gives us confidence and courage, removes our inhibitions, relieves boredom and stress, eases pain, helps us to relax, and releases the imagination.'[1] By the time we're old enough to drink we've probably received these pro-alcohol messages thousands and thousands of times. So deeply have they been absorbed into our brains, it's no surprise we end up believing that alcohol is the perfect accompaniment to human life. Annie Grace, author of the powerful *This Naked Mind: Control alcohol, find freedom, discover happiness and change your life*, says it's instilled from birth: 'Like most things that have been ingrained in us since childhood, we believe in alcohol without question, like we believe the sky is blue.'[2]

Pro-drinking messages are reinforced over and over again in our customs and rituals. So many milestones, moments and points of connection are synonymous with alcohol. Births, deaths and marriages—arguably the big three in terms of milestones—have strong associations with drink that go back centuries.

Weddings are boozy even before the big day arrives—aren't hen and stag parties all about getting the bride and groom monumentally hammered? Someone I know was pushed to drink so much at her hen party that she had to go off to the toilet in the middle to vomit before she could continue on. She confided later that she hadn't actually wanted to get so drunk, but felt expected to do so. Wedding days themselves often feature copious amounts of booze, and many happy couples would be foolish not to factor a huge booze spend into their budget. I can't tell you the number of times I've got wasted at a wedding. I even treated my own like a massive, debauched party. We ran out of alcohol halfway through the night and someone had to go on an emergency booze run. The next day I was so sleep-deprived and hungover I could barely talk.

A new baby entering the world is also often celebrated with a drink. 'Wetting the baby's head' used to mean delicately sprinkling holy water over a newborn's crown, but nowadays it tends to denote consuming large amounts of grog (or, according to *Urban Dictionary*, having 'a drinking spree'). Funerals can also be very liquid affairs. Once the ceremony is over and the tears have been wiped, it's time to drink up large. They don't call it 'drowning your sorrows' for nothing.

We've taken this notion of raising a glass on special occasions and widened it out beyond births, deaths and marriages. As neuroscientist and recovering addict Judith Grisel brilliantly puts it in her book *Never Enough: The neuroscience and experience of addiction*: 'Social convention is pickled in the intoxicating juice of alcohol.'[3] Celebrating a birthday, graduating university, landing a job, getting engaged, buying a house, selling a house, gaining a promotion, marking an anniversary—all of these are seen as a good reason to drink. Christmas, New Year's Eve, the Super Bowl, All Blacks' test matches—these too. Friday and Saturday nights, of course. Farewelling a colleague, thanking your kid's sports coach, saying 'I'm sorry'—all often done with a gift of alcohol. It truly has become ubiquitous in the business of being alive.

So deeply ingrained is our belief in alcohol as a good thing and a vital ingredient in life that even when it's dragging us down we struggle to see how life will be fun without it. When I was at the end of my drinking days, utterly miserable and low, one of the biggest things I had to contend with was imagining my future with no alcohol in it. Despite the clear evidence that it was doing me so much harm, I was utterly terrified that life without wine would be dreadful and boring. Even though I was having no fun with it, I was terrified that there'd be no fun without it—it was madness! But that's purely as a result of the deep cultural indoctrination I'd received regarding alcohol, and the crazily pro-drinking, booze-saturated nature of my environment. I'd picture the years ahead littered with special occasions rendered worthless and dull. I imagined myself sitting like a lame duck in the corner at gatherings, sober and miserable while everyone else partied away merrily with a drink in their hand. I imagined myself wound up like a top every Friday night, unable to unwind with a drink. I imagined myself bereft at my children's weddings, unable to toast the happy couple with a glass full of champagne. I imagined myself sitting on the balcony of fancy five-star hotels in tropical locations (I was aiming high with my imaginary future), glum because I wasn't able to celebrate the moment with a glistening glass of chardonnay. These fears were real, and they're felt by many others. As Belinda admits in her story shared later on page 84: 'It was this feeling that if I didn't have the alcohol, I was missing out on the next level of fun.' And as Veronica confessed in the previous chapter: 'It is a struggle imagining how to live sober and still enjoy my life.'

But if you stop to properly unpick these beliefs, as authors like Annie Grace and Allen Carr have done exhaustively in their very powerful books, you'll see what a crock of shit they truly are. Properly relaxing is about a million things, such as putting on comfy clothes, tucking away your phone, being with friends, walking the dog, lighting a scented candle, getting a head massage, reading a good book, insert your own genuinely relaxing activity here . . . not drinking a brain-numbing liquid. Parties are about getting together with people you love, feeling fabulous in a new pair of shoes, sharing a laugh with friends, meeting new and interesting people, eating yummy nibbles . . . not imbibing a substance that messes with your emotions. Weddings are about witnessing a public declaration of love, hearing moving speeches, eating delicious food and dancing the night away . . . not sinking so much piss you end up slurring your words and falling over. And sitting on the balcony of a fancy five-star hotel in a tropical location is . . .

well, it's sitting on the balcony of a goddam fancy five-star hotel in a tropical location! Hello?! Why does what liquid you have in your glass have the power to make that moment, or any other moment, milestone or point of human connection worthwhile? There are so many other factors that contribute to good, fun and meaningful times. But that's not what we tend to believe given all the pro-drinking messages we receive from birth, or what our booze-soaked environment is telling us. No wonder we're fearful when faced with the prospect of quitting. As Helidth Ravenholm and Carole Reid once said, 'Human cultures are hugely guilty of "it is done this way" behaviour.'[4] But, just because we've always done something one way, doesn't mean we can't turn it around. I'm living proof of that, as are many thousands of others.

4.

Olivia

'I think it's self-care, but actually
it's the opposite of self-care.'

There was always alcohol around me growing up. I'm one of five kids and we'd always be down at the local social club with Mum and Dad and all their friends, cruising around drinking Coke, eating crisps, falling asleep on the bench seats and getting bundled into the car after dark. There was always alcohol in the house as well. When I was about fifteen we started taxing the liquor cabinet and making rocket fuel. At around seventeen we'd pretend to be asleep then put a pillow or towel in the bed, sneak out the back and go joyriding. Some friends across town could drive and they'd come and pick us up in their parents' cars. I remember going to a party and getting so drunk I fell back and banged my head on a tennis court. I guess that's the start of the memories—or lack of memories—of binge drinking.

I left school and got a job at a law firm as an office junior. Friday-night drinks were always a big thing—they were free and it was non-stop. On the weekends I'd drink lots of beer with my boyfriend and his mates. When I was about 22 I got a job as a cycle courier. Not too much drinking went down then—we were all a bit lightweight because we were so super fit. That's when I started getting into other stuff besides alcohol, like weed and acid and stuff.

I moved to the UK and lived there for ten years, drinking a lot of beer, partying a lot and taking a lot of Class A drugs. So much of everything, every weekend. I met some wonderful people and went to some great festivals. The jobs were all right, never too taxing on my brain, hence why I could party at the same time. Sometimes my group of friends, we'd say, 'we're not drinking this week', then we'd be on the train home and someone would go, 'I need a pint', and then we'd all end up at the pub at the train station. One pint would turn into five—you know the drill—and this is just on a Monday night. So much for the alcohol-free week. I got into some dangerous situations. One time I fell asleep on the top level of a night bus after a drunken night out and woke up just as the bus was driving into the terminal. I walked down the stairs and the driver said, 'Where did you come from?!' He had just finished his run and was going to cash up. He ended up giving me a ride home.

I was in my late twenties when drinking came up as a thing I should maybe address. I went to see a hypnotherapist to try and quit cigarettes and worked out drinking was the trigger for the smoking, and it was actually the drinking that I needed to stop. But there was no way that was going to happen—we were having too much fun. My mental health was a bit up and down at times though. I'm prone to depression, and drinking and taking drugs definitely didn't help. I probably should have been dealing with how I was feeling underneath instead.

After a decade in the UK I came home and was here for a year, during which time my dad died. That was terribly traumatic. He had a heart attack and survived it, but picked up an infection in hospital that killed him. That was nine years ago and I still think about it daily.

His death triggered me to drink more and I suffered quite bad depression. I was working in a café and I wasn't good, wasn't doing well at all. I see photos of me around that time and I'd lost so much weight. I was just trying to blur it all out.

I met my husband at a gig—he plays in a band. He was a big drinker when we first met, and we used to drink so much red wine together. After the kids came along we had a rule at first that we wouldn't drink until after they'd gone to bed, but that didn't last. My general habit nowadays is to have a couple of beers while cooking the kids' dinner, and then maybe two glasses of wine. That's every single day. I think it's self-care, but actually it's the opposite of self-care. It's slowing me down and fuzzing my mind. And there's still a lot of binging in my circle of friends. We'll go out dancing at a nightclub and we'll preload. And then we'll go and spend a fortune on drinks that we don't even need.

Just lately my husband has quit drinking. He first stopped for two weeks, then a month, then he said he was feeling so good he wasn't going to drink at all ever again. He's replaced the alcohol with eating well and doing yoga—lifestyle stuff. It was pretty casual for him compared to my inner dialogue about it. I've been wrestling with myself about alcohol for about five years, just feeling like I'm not in control. Last year I stopped drinking for a while because I wasn't feeling good. My clothes were all tight, my mind was all foggy. I was going to stop for a month but only made it to 26 days. Afterwards I almost started drinking more.

Right now I'm almost at the end of another stint off. It's taken almost a whole month to stop thinking about not having a drink. I wouldn't say the cravings have gone, but during those first couple of weeks I was thinking, *Actually I'm much better when I drink.* Because I was getting even more tense, yelling at the kids more. And my mental health has been a bit up and down. So I was thinking, *If I had a drink I could calm down.* But I know that if you give anything up there's an adjustment period and you've got to ride through it. The best thing has been awesome sleeps. I've got this app called 'I Am Sober', and it tells me how much money and time I've saved by not drinking. It also sends me little teachings and motivations every day. So far I've saved $450! I'm going to spend it this weekend: we're going to Sydney to see The Cure play at the Opera House. That'll be the end of my stint off because I couldn't do that and not drink, not with the people I'm going with. I'm hoping that I come back and maybe leave alcohol for special occasions, and I'll try not to have it in the house, but I've said that before. Given how good I'm feeling right now, I'd like to become a sensible drinker. I'd like to appreciate it rather than abuse it. If I can't be a sensible drinker, I'm probably going to have to quit.

5.

Bonding agent

One of the most startling aspects of alcohol's ubiquity in our society today is the way that it has inserted itself firmly in the middle of the glorious natural phenomenon that is female bonding. There's a lot to love about being a woman, but one of the best things of all is that it gives you automatic entry into the girl club, a glorious place where you get to connect with and be lifted up by other women. Whether it's the bestie you connect with almost daily, the colleague you share your lunch breaks with, the friend with whom you take weekly dog walks, your old mate back in your home town, the buddy down the street, your once-a-month book club, your Friday-night gang or those dear old friends you organise special trips away with, females rely on girlfriends to balance out and enrich our lives. Girlfriends help us unpick our emotions, make sense of other people and gain clarity on the world. As Jacqueline Mroz says in her book *Girl Talk: What science can tell us about female friendship*, 'We tell our friends secrets that we wouldn't entrust to anyone else; we cry on their shoulders when things have gone wrong and we toast them when they've succeeded; we talk to them about our significant others, our kids, our parents; we go on adventures together; and we laugh over each other's imperfections. What would we do without our friends?'[1]

I don't know what I would do without my girlfriends; they are a hugely important part of my life. They listen to me, support me and care about me, as I do them. Some I communicate with weekly, some monthly, some only once or twice a year (and that's okay too). We meet in person, call each other on the phone, text, email and group message. We can always sense when it's been too long and some sort of a catch-up or get-together is needed. And what do we do when we connect? We talk. We talk and we talk and we talk. We talk about what we're working on and what we're involved in. We talk about our families, our colleagues, our kids and our parents. We talk about pop culture, the royal family, politics and social injustices. We talk about our periods, beauty, fashion and food. And we talk about our emotions, how we're feeling, what we're processing, our dreams, hopes and fears. It's awesome and I love it all.

There's something particularly unique, special and important about female friendships, according to Mroz, something that is quite different from male friendships or relationships with our family members. 'We feel better when we're with our friends—even knowing they're there for us can make us happy. And research has begun to back up the magic of friendship and its connection to our health. Having friends improves our immunity, promotes healing, lowers blood pressure, and makes us feel less depressed—it even makes us live longer.'[2] Mroz interviewed many women for *Girl Talk*, curious to know what values they most looked for in a girlfriend. She found that the two most important qualities women are after in a friend are emotional support and authenticity. Other qualities mentioned were loyalty, success, being a good listener, compassion, intelligence, humour, optimism and trustworthiness. No one in her study mentioned 'drinking alcohol together' as a vital component of a successful friendship. So why is that so often what we do?

Drinking together has become one of our most common pastimes: socialising with sauvignon, bonding over bubbles or gossiping with gin. Girls' trips are usually always planned with drinking at the centre of them—just take a good look around social media and you'll find endless photos of women celebrating wild nights out on holiday weekends, or sipping cocktails on the beach together in exotic locations. The boozy girls' trip is immortalised in many Hollywood movies (see *Bridesmaids, Girls Trip, Rough Night, Wine Country*), and speakers events for women are often planned with alcohol front and centre. ('Bubbles and Inspiration' showcases alcohol's involvement in the name and 'Broad-ly Speaking' is sponsored by more than one liquor company, with drinks included in the ticket price.) Many of our more intimate clubs and groups also often seem to be centred on drinking. Writing at addiction.com, Megan Peters claims most book clubs are actually 'midweek socializing freed from scrutiny by the pretense of an intellectual discussion that mostly never happens',[3] a fact that's been backed up by more than one woman who has confided in me that their all-female book clubs are really just an excuse to get together and drink wine.

(Not all female book clubs are like that, I hasten to add!)

So what is it we're after when we drink together? Are we looking for a way to elevate our experiences together and strengthen our bonds? In her 2019 research paper '"I feel like I have to become part of that identity": Negotiating femininities and friendships through alcohol consumption in Newcastle, UK', Emily Nicholls found that alcohol was often used by women as a tool, 'albeit at times an unpredictable and unwieldy one', to enhance socialising and to establish trust and intimacy in ways that cement friendships. She also discovered that women tended to focus on the positive aspects of going out and drinking with their friends, even when the night ended in messy, drunken drama. 'For several of the participants, the messy, embodied consequences of intoxication—"crying for an hour", losing the ability to get home safely or even vomiting in public—were not framed as problematic, but rather as further opportunities for bonding and intimacy.'[4] So is that what it is? We like drinking together so that we can look after one another when we fall apart? Is the definition of a good friend someone who will hold your hair back while you vomit?

When researching this book I heard time and again from women whose friend groups were focused almost entirely on drinking together. Single mum Grace, who shares her story later on page 48, said getting drunk with her 'big, boozy social group' was 'just the lifestyle; it's how we catch up'. The fear of losing these friends is a big reason why she's hesitant to stop drinking. Same goes for Veronica, who on page 30 told us about her boozy social group in the city after living in an isolated rural area for years. 'I fear losing that if I'm not drinking,' she said.

There's no denying that getting drunk with your friends can be an awesome, fun experience (goodness knows I did it for years before the wheels fell off my habit), and there are studies clearly showing that there are social and well-being benefits to be derived from drinking alcohol in relaxed social environments.[5] But does alcohol need to be front and centre of every type of girly bonding experience or female gathering? Do we need alcohol to give currency to all our social catch-ups? Is wine the foundation of a deep, lasting friendship? Or is it all those other values and qualities that Jacqueline Mroz discovered in her research, things like authenticity and being a good listener? Is it possible that alcohol, rather than connecting us like we think it does, actually serves to push us apart?

Laura thinks it does. She's a lively, sociable city girl who struggled to find friends after moving to a new country. Stuck at home feeling lonely and bored one day, she decided to reach out via Facebook to connect with other women in her community. 'I created a social group for mums to meet mums. The whole goal was to get people who are fairly isolated, maybe people that are new to town, to get them out and about to meet other people in a really relaxed atmosphere.'

She began organising events, hiring venues, sorting out themes and giveaways. 'I disguised it a little bit as going out for shared plates and dinner, but really it was about going out and finding drinking buddies to have fun with and party.' Her idea took off: many women came along and everyone appeared to be having a great time, but by the third or fourth event Laura said she realised the alcohol, while good for fast-tracking a sense of connection, was actually making it all rather hollow. 'Once you've got your beer or wine goggles on, everyone's a friend, aren't they? Because essentially drinking just brings the truth serum out and you end up telling your life story to someone you actually don't know or potentially don't even like. We think it's a social thing that connects us, but it's such bullshit.'

She gently cut her ties with the group and worked instead on connecting with women in different ways—going for walks and sharing activities with their kids. 'I have got new friends now, and we get together over coffee. It's lovely, and we have really honest conversations. I don't want to be the fun police. I mean, there's a time and a place for going to a bar. But are you going to really get to know somebody over a margarita?'

6.

Grace

'We talk about how crap our weeks
have been while we get drunk.'

I grew up overseas, and my parents aren't big drinkers, so there wasn't a huge amount of alcohol around in my childhood. There was no drinking age where we lived, so we had the odd drink around the age of thirteen, fourteen, but it wasn't until I came back to New Zealand aged sixteen that I started binge drinking. I think I was trying to be cool and fit in. New Zealand was a bit of a culture shock for me, just a different sort of scene. It was no longer cool to be in school—in New Zealand it was heaps cooler to be out drinking and smoking pot and cigarettes.

Once I started partying I was always the biggest drinker, a real party girl. I only ever drank to get drunk, but I seemed to always be able to hold it together. I've always been quite functional and I've never woken up in someone's bed and thought, *Oh no, how did I end up here?* But I am very susceptible to having blackouts. I often don't remember things—it's common. There used to be whole bars that I don't remember going to. When I was at uni I would sometimes wake up in the morning and have to ring all my friends to try and find out where my car was. Like, I would have no idea where I had last driven to. So we'd all have to do a bit of investigating and try to figure out which streets to walk around to try and find my car. We thought it was funny.

I ended up working in Europe in my twenties, and that was probably when I started drinking every day. It was a real work hard, play hard environment. I met my husband overseas and we eventually moved back to New Zealand, bought a house, got married and had a son. That was probably a period in my life that was not hugely boozy. My husband's not a big drinker, so during that time I'd just have a couple of wines every evening. That's how I drink if I'm not at a social occasion—just a relaxing couple of glasses at the end of the day.

We ended up breaking up, but I wasn't too upset about it. It felt like a good thing for me. I felt like I found myself again. I wanted to have a good time and meet new people, so I started going out and partying again. After a couple of years I met this guy and we ended up moving in together. He was a very heavy drinker and we would get really drunk together all the time. Everything we did involved alcohol. Any occasion, even going to the beach, would involve a bottle of wine. We socialised a lot and we'd often have a huge night, be the last to leave, and then when we got home we would carry on drinking.

I started getting worried. I said to my partner, 'I think we've got a drinking problem and we should try and cut back a bit,' but he dismissed me. I mentioned to my friends that I thought I had a problem and needed to cut back. They wanted to support me, but the way they did that was by not seeing me. They'd be like, 'Oh, don't ask Grace—she's trying not to drink.'

I stopped drinking for a while before the end of the relationship. During that period people just stopped asking me out. I didn't see anyone. I think people felt judged and that's why they didn't want to hang out with me. I wasn't preaching about it, but it was confronting for them and they didn't like it. They'd say, 'Oh, God, you're not going to get all righteous on us, are you?' I had to pretend that I was drinking alcohol because it was easier.

I split from my partner a few years ago. It was traumatic emotionally—still is. I'm not quite through it. A big part of why I left him was the drinking, but the really weird thing is that I'm now drinking the most I ever have—more than when we were together.

My close friends are all drinkers—we're in a big, boozy social group. It's just the lifestyle; it's how we catch up. By Wednesday everyone is messaging each other saying, 'God, I need a drink', trying to get together so we can talk about how crap our weeks have been while we get drunk. It's kind of weird, especially given we're all quite health-conscious. Everyone goes to the gym and runs and does yoga.

I'll go out of my way to create social circumstances. It'll be Sunday afternoon and I'll want a wine, and I'll be texting just about every person I know, saying, 'Come over for a glass of wine.' I can have parties at home alone too. I drank a bottle of wine at home here on Friday night, watching a movie with my son. It's really easy to do, and I won't even feel drunk. That just touches the sides. If I'm going somewhere and know there's not going to be any alcohol there I'll quickly down a couple of glasses of wine at home beforehand. I once poured wine into a takeaway coffee cup when taking my son to music lessons, so I could sit in the car and have a drink while I waited. I remember thinking, *God, this is wrong.*

Often I think maybe I'll have a couple of nights off but I never do. I had to travel away for work the other day. We finished at five o'clock and had to be at the airport to fly home at six. When we got to the airport they didn't sell wine at the domestic terminal. I was just beside myself. I was so horrified, quite distraught about it.

I am cringing sometimes now and I feel guilty. When I have a big night, I wake up and I really don't like myself. I get so angry if I've wasted half my weekend with hangovers. I can't do things properly with my son, and he seems to know. One day he said something to me about going to the movies and I said, 'What movie? You never told me—you can't just go. You gotta ask.' And he said, 'I did ask you last night,' and I said 'Did you?' and he said, 'You were probably drunk.' And I thought, *That's not cool for my child to say that.* Things like that are red flags.

I would like to improve my relationship with alcohol. My problem is that once I get to a certain point I just keep going until I can't remember anything. It's like a switch has been flicked. I wish I could just have a good time and go home.

I don't want to get to the point where I have to not drink. I feel like I'd miss out on a lot. And it's fun. I enjoy wine, I enjoy cocktails. I actually like the flavour of it. And I like going to vineyards, all of that. So I'm just trying to keep tabs on myself.

7.

How did we get here?

It wasn't always like this, you know. We didn't always live in a booze-soaked society where alcohol was granted such a privileged position. We didn't always rely so wholeheartedly on alcohol as a means of relaxation and celebration. And drink certainly didn't use to be so firmly inserted into the rituals of female bonding. I think it really pays to remember this—that the status quo of today with regard to alcohol is particular to this point in time. There have been many other realities over the years, accompanied by much debate and various attempts at control and regulation. This is true of all the Western countries that have fully embraced alcohol, but I'm just going to talk about New Zealand here, because that's where I live.

In my beloved little country, population under 5 million, we didn't have any alcohol until around 200 years ago, unlike Turkey, for example, where they've found evidence of alcohol dating back over 10,000 years. It wasn't until the early 1800s that alcohol arrived in New Zealand, brought here by the first European settlers. Most of them were single men, and they moved around the country working in remote areas, pissing it up large in centralised settlements on their days off. There was a lot of drunken debauchery and general bad behaviour, which lawmakers at the time tried to get under control with the passing of loads of laws and regulations—almost 50 at one count, including things like no selling liquor to the indigenous Māori population, no dancing girls in bars and no distilling of spirits.

When more European women began arriving here in the second half of the 1800s and family life became more established, a feisty temperance movement emerged that lobbied hard against liquor for many decades (the temperance movement is still regarded as one of New Zealand's most powerful and sustained public movements ever). The temperance movement wanted to curb liquor sales and keep intakes low and harm to a minimum. Those on the other side of the coin—alcohol producers, hoteliers and so on—were, in contrast, keen to see liquor sales grow, so they also banded together to form a lobby group. And so began a fairly even tussle between the two sides. (Take note of the phrase 'a fairly even tussle', because *spoiler alert*, times have changed.) Over the next century or so the temperance movement and the booze lobby went head to head to try to get their interests met. Each side worked hard to sway public opinion through media campaigns and the like, and to lobby and influence elected officials to pass laws in their favour.

One early success of the temperance movement was an Act called the Local Option Poll, which prevented any new liquor outlets from being opened in a community unless the majority of local residents supported it. It stated that, any time someone wanted to start selling alcohol, ratepayers in the area had to be polled to see if they were keen or not. Imagine that! Such a huge contrast from today, when practically any man and his dog can get a licence, and if residents aren't keen they have to put in a huge amount of time and effort opposing it. Other restrictive regulations that went through were a 10 p.m. closing time, a purchasing age of 21 and no women allowed to work in bars. In 1916 there was even a War Regulation Amendment that prohibited drinkers from shouting rounds. (It was roundly ignored.)

One of the most fundamental laws of all, in terms of its long-term impact on New Zealanders' drinking habits, was the 1917 Sale of Liquor Restriction Act, which stated that all licensed establishments had to close at 6 p.m. It was meant to be a temporary war-time thing, but ended up staying in place for 50 years! The temperance movement lobbied hard for it, and interestingly the liquor industry did little to oppose it. They saw it as a good way to remove some of the power and urgency of the temperance movement (which worked), and they suspected that the men (and it *was* mostly men) in bars would just drink faster and harder to get the same amount of liquor in them in a shorter amount of time. They were right. So began what was referred to as the 'six o'clock swill'—the practice of men crowding together in huge beer barns to drink as much alcohol as they could as fast as they could before the place closed. This practice—which went on for 50 years, don't forget!—is often blamed for being one of the biggest contributing factors to our current 'hard and fast' drinking culture.[1]

Fast-forward to today and it's common practice in New Zealand for people to head out for the night with the explicit intention of getting drunk. (I spent most of my twenties doing exactly that.) And we have no issue with displaying our extreme drunkenness in public, either. As the authors of *Pleasure, Profit and Pain: Alcohol in New Zealand and the contemporary culture of intoxication* put it: 'Our contemporary culture of intoxication accepts and celebrates the exhibition of drunken behaviour. There is minimal social shame associated with public displays of intoxication including vomiting, loss of bodily control, loss of memory and passing out.'[2]

Six o'clock closing eventually ended in 1967, and over the next twenty years or so that previously mentioned 'fairly even tussle' between the pro- and anti-liquor lobbies slowly morphed into a very uneven contest. Liquor licences became easier to come by, closing time moved later and the drinking age was lowered. And then, in 1989, right about the time I was being kicked out of my high-school graduation for being drunk, we got the most monumental, game-changing law of them all—the Sale and Supply of Liquor Act. This is the law that opened the floodgates for alcohol in this country and changed everything. Sunday trading was allowed, as was 24-hour trading. Liquor licences were simplified into just two types—on-licences (you drink where the alcohol is purchased) and off-licences (you can take it away). The number and type of on-licences permitted was expanded and the criteria for getting them was simplified, and supermarkets and grocery stores were granted off-licences, allowing them to sell wine (beer came later). As a result the number of licences issued expanded rapidly—doubling, tripling, and then some. At the time of the law change we had 4000 liquor licences; currently we have just under 12,000.

Grant Hewison is a lawyer who has spent many hours over the past five years helping community groups oppose liquor licences in their areas. He told me they're fighting a losing battle. 'The industry is now so embedded in our communities, closing existing liquor stores is almost impossible. Stopping new ones from opening is also extremely difficult, and in my experience over the last five years we've lost more than we've won.' Hewison believes allowing booze into supermarkets has had one of the most profound impacts on our drinking culture. 'One of the really perverse things about the sale of alcohol in supermarkets is that it's inevitably right next to the fruit and veggie section. So you come into your supermarket and there's your fruit and vegetables, and right next to them is your alcohol section, with all the brightly coloured advertising that goes with that. It's not only normalising it but really entices and encourages you to purchase. And our duopoly supermarkets sell alcohol at very cheap prices.'

After the 1989 law change, in addition to a huge jump in liquor licences, production of alcohol (wine in particular) also exploded, marketing (to women and young people especially) took off, sales skyrocketed, consumption levels soared and buckets and buckets of money was pumped into the liquor industry's coffers. One public-health campaigner likens any attempt to fight against alcohol's place in our society to being put in a ring against Muhammad Ali 'with both legs hobbled and one arm tied behind your back'. What were the lawmakers who designed this hugely pro-booze Act thinking? I can tell you what they were thinking. They were thinking neoliberal thoughts of deregulation and a free market (à la Reagan and Thatcher). They were thinking less state control of alcohol, letting the liquor industry regulate itself. And they were thinking that loosening restrictions would normalise alcohol, which would lead us to become a nation of moderate, sophisticated drinkers. Look how well that turned out.

It's currently estimated that alcohol is causing around $7 billion worth of harm every year in lost labour production, health costs, road crashes, crime, deaths and reduced quality of life.[3] Around 800 New Zealanders die due to alcohol every year, from injuries, cancer and other chronic diseases,[4] and 70,000 alcohol-related physical and sexual assaults are recorded.[5] Of the 80 per cent of adults who drink, at least a quarter of those do so to hazardous levels. Excessive alcohol consumption is a major risk factor for suicide and it contributes to around a third of all road-accident deaths. One in four admissions to hospital emergency departments is alcohol-related, and our police receive over 70,000 calls a year involving booze. Between 600 and 3000 babies are born with Fetal Alcohol Spectrum Disorder in this country each year.[6] These are just the stats for New Zealand; the situation is similarly dire in other places like Australia, the United States and much of Europe. Globally, the World Health Organization estimates that 3.3 million people die every year because of excessive alcohol use.

Here in New Zealand, police, doctors, social workers, public-health advocates, medical officers of health, psychiatrists, university professors, the Cancer Society and alcohol action campaigners are all crying out for changes to be made to our liquor laws. But to date they've been largely ignored. A Law Commission report and a Government Inquiry into

Mental Health and Addiction have both recommended widespread changes to our alcohol regulations, but they're not being listened to either. Some tinkering has been done around the edges: in 2012 the Sale and Supply of Alcohol Act came in (to replace the bombshell 1989 Act) but it didn't do anything about the biggest three aspects of alcohol regulation that research has proved makes all the difference—price, availability and marketing.[7] I'm not sure how strong the chances are of any government making changes to those three things given alcohol reform is seen as political suicide—thanks largely to the rhetoric pushed by the alcohol lobby.

With only a small and underfunded lobby group arguing for the public-health side of things, and a lack of any political will to put in tighter regulations, it seems as though there's little chance of the current situation changing. Hewison certainly isn't hopeful. 'It's not a happy state of affairs. The alcohol industry is extraordinarily dominant. Through our neoliberal policies we've empowered them with enormous wealth, and they use that to influence our politicians—mostly covertly, but overtly as well. They lobby, actively, day in day out, politicians from all parties and spectrums, to maintain that wealth. Not just maintain it, but increase it.'

8.

Mandy

'At the back of my mind is this nagging thought of, Is this another tobacco?'

I think my upbringing was pretty low-key in terms of alcohol. I don't remember it being around much unless my parents had a party on, or it was a special occasion like Easter or Christmas. At fifteen a family friend offered me a glass of wine with mum and dad present and they didn't say no. I think they took the view that one glass when you were about that age wasn't going to be a massive problem. Around that age my friends started getting older brothers or sisters to buy booze and bring it into town so we could meet up and drink it. I never actually did that, but later on I went to some parties—maybe I was sixteen by then—where someone had done a booze run and bought some bottles of wine. It was kind of fun and exciting, but whether that was the wine or the whole thing of sneaking drinks, I don't know.

I was always conscious of not losing control. I didn't throw up drinking alcohol until I was eighteen or nineteen, and then only once. I had the knowledge drilled into me in school health classes of what could happen if you did lose control. It was about safety as a woman and not putting yourself at risk or you could end up with someone doing something to you. I guess I didn't want to put myself in a situation where I wasn't in control of myself. So I drank just enough to have a bit of a buzz but not to go past that. I'm still conscious of that. There's a line where I'm like, *That's enough. Don't have any more, because you'll regret it.*

I left school and went to university to study law. I probably drank quite a lot while I was studying, but I was always careful and controlled, conscious of other things that I wanted to do. It was expensive too and I didn't have the money. I wasn't going to draw down my whole student loan and spend it all on having a good time.

When I was close to finishing my law degree, the big law firms all came to the campus to try and persuade the graduates they were interested in to come and work for them. They flew down to interview senior law students, but before they did the interviews they held a cocktail party to wine and dine us. So our first meeting of these lawyers and HR people who were coming to interview us was at a cocktail party. I think we were all very aware that we had to be kind of grown up, but equally—free booze! I had more than one offer from more than one law firm so I got flown to where they were all based, and wined and dined some more. It was amazing. I felt like I'd worked hard, and I deserved this glamorous lifestyle that was coming my way. I was taken out to all these top restaurants night after night after night. I remember thinking, *I don't think I can take any more of this food and wine.* I just felt revolting by the end of it.

I don't think you would have been judged harshly for not drinking, but at the same time, if you are out bonding with people who are going to give you work, you could say that it helped to be a drinker. I never saw anybody in a situation where I thought there was a power imbalance or anything like that, but I've heard plenty of stories and I definitely had the sense that it was unhealthy at times, because there was alcohol everywhere. Some people would get quite drunk and sloppy. It wasn't frowned upon at all, but you knew that if you really misbehaved it would be bad. If anyone was in a really risky position, I think there would have been people who would have stepped in, but the general vibe was just having fun.

I worked in law firms for years and we always had Friday-night drinks in the office bar. There was supposed to be a partner in charge of the bar at all times, but I don't think that was always the case. I'm much further on in my career now and have moved out of law firms, but from what I understand they've taken a good look at themselves lately and are more careful around alcohol. I have heard anecdotally that they've changed some of their practices—limiting Friday-night drinks to just two hours long, doing social activities that aren't focused on drinking, things like that.

My work now still involves a lot of socialising. Some weeks I might drink every single night at functions. I won't drink too much on each occasion, but I'm probably still drinking too much overall. I once saw the Ministry of Health guidelines for recommended drinking levels and went, 'Oh! They're quite low!' So I try and keep that in mind and count how many glasses I've had. It's hard at functions when they come around and top you up constantly. Expensive restaurants will do that a lot—come around and top you up when you've got half a glass left—so it's easy to lose count. I'm very aware of that and stop them from doing it. I'll make them wait till I've finished before I let them top me up, just so I can know how many glasses I'm drinking. There are definitely weeks where if I've got a lot of work functions on I'd be blasting the recommended limit out of the water, and that's not very good. But I'm not really worried because I'll think, *Whoa, okay. Maybe next week I'll have none.* It'd be really difficult, I think, if you were battling with alcohol because it's everywhere.

I will have a drink at home at five o'clock some days, but it's not every day and I try not to during the week. If I buy a bottle of wine or two at the start of the week with the groceries, once it's gone, it's gone. I wouldn't go and buy more. I'm quite a disciplined person. In my head I would ideally not drink more than a bottle, ever, in a sitting and usually I try not to drink more than two or three glasses in one night. If I've had a rough day and I'm stressed I might come home and have two glasses, and then that'll be it. I'd happily stop. I've read that if you meditate and do yoga, and go for walks and exercise more, or whatever, those things will help you relax better. So, even if I might feel like I'd rather just sit on the couch and have a couple of wines, logic tells me that it's not going to help, even if in the short term it feels better.

It has crossed my mind that it might be healthier to

get alcohol right out of my life, but I don't really want to. I don't like the taste of fizzy drink, so I can't substitute it for a Coke or something because I don't like that. I do like the taste of a wine and I don't want to be a non-drinker. I also don't think I drink so much that it's a problem. I'm in control of it and I like it. I don't want it out of my life, but I don't want it to take over either.

At the back of my mind is this nagging thought of, *Is this another tobacco?* That in 50 years time people are gonna look back and laugh, like we laugh now at those ads that used to say, 'Your doctor recommends cigarettes.' Doctors recommended it! 'Have a cigarette a day and it will make you healthy.' I wonder if we will look back at how we're treating alcohol now and say, 'Oh, my God. What were we doing?' We're effectively pouring poison down our throats. Maybe we should all be looking at it, no matter how much we like the taste.

Part Two

WHAT IT'S DOING TO US

9.

It's all about dopamine

In her book *Never Enough: The neuroscience and experience of addiction*, Judith Grisel describes addiction as 'a merciless compulsion to remodel experience by altering brain function'.[1] She's talking about full-blown addiction (hence the 'merciless compulsion'), but the 'remodel experience by altering brain function' part applies to everyone when they drink alcohol. That's what we're doing. When we say we're 'taking the edge off' what we're actually saying is that we want to alter our brain function. When we claim to 'need a drink' what we're actually saying is, 'I need to shift my reality.' I have had the odd person try to tell me the only reason they drink alcohol is for the taste, but I've always been a bit sceptical about that claim given it's impossible to separate the taste of alcohol from the effect of it. If it really was only about the taste then why not drink alcohol-free wine and beer? No, the bottom line is that it's the effect of alcohol that makes it so alluring. If you gave a toddler a sippy cup filled with whisky they wouldn't slurp it down; they'd toss it aside in disgust. But as adults we grow to tolerate—enjoy, even—the taste of alcohol because of the association we've made with how it affects us. And the way it affects us comes from a complex series of scientific processes and reactions.

First of all, I just want to be clear about what we're talking about when we say 'alcohol', because there are actually three different types of alcohol: isopropyl, methyl and ethyl. Isopropyl is found in cleaning products and antiseptics. Methyl is used as the basis for things like antifreeze and paint stripper (and it can make you go blind if you drink it, so don't). Ethyl alcohol is the one we humans commonly drink; when we talk about 'alcohol', we're talking about ethyl alcohol, also known as ethanol.

Ethyl alcohol is made through a process of fermentation, where yeast is used to convert the sugars in grains, fruits and vegetables. Most wines come from fermented grapes, most beers come from fermented malted barley, and different types of spirits come from a huge variety of fermented fruits and veggies (for example, juniper berries for gin, or potatoes for vodka). Many different additives are added to the basic fermented product to create different varietals, flavours and types of alcoholic drinks. I couldn't even begin to count all the different alcohols on offer in the world right now. Suffice it to say, there are a lot.

When you put alcohol into your body, first your mouth and tongue absorb a little bit through small blood vessels, then it goes to your stomach, where some gets absorbed depending on how much food is there. Most of it moves through to the small intestine, and it's from there that it travels into the blood. The blood then carries it all over the body—brain, heart, lungs, limbs, liver, kidneys and all the rest. Some alcohol is breathed out through the lungs (that's why breathalysers work and booze breath is a thing), some is excreted out as sweat through the skin (euw), and some is urinated out thanks to the kidneys. Most of the alcohol you put into your body is broken down by the liver. It's a slow process, as the liver can only filter a certain amount at a time; that is, one standard drink per hour.

Ah, the old 'standard drink' thing. Let's pause here on the science for a moment. Who can say off the top of their heads exactly what a standard drink is? We just don't tend to deal in those measurements in our day-to-day lives. Standard drink measures are mostly used by people in the health and addiction sectors for things like measuring safe versus hazardous drinking levels, or recommending daily and weekly limits.

Exactly how many standard drinks are contained within a bottle, cask or can is usually listed on the label, but I'm fairly certain most of us don't read the fine print. I certainly never did. When measuring a standard drink it's all about the amount of 'pure alcohol' contained within, which is why the amount differs for different types and strengths of alcohol (another reason why it's so hard to get a handle on). Just to lay it out: one standard drink is 10 grams of pure alcohol. So one standard drink of a spirit that is 42 per cent proof is 30 millilitres, for an average-strength beer (4 per cent) it's 330 millilitres, and for wine that is 12.5 per cent it's 100 millilitres.[2] Right before I quit drinking (when I was busy trying to sort myself out) I discovered what a standard drink was and went straight away to measure 100 millilitres of wine using my red plastic kitchen measuring cup. I then poured that into my usual wine glass and was shocked to discover that my 'one glass of wine' was actually more than three and a half standard drinks (yes, I used enormous wine glasses, and yes, I poured buckets). I then read that a binge for women is considered to be four or more standard drinks in two hours. I did the math on that one as well and realised I was binging basically every night. I used to think binge meant 'drink till you vomit', but no. Anyhoo . . . back to the science.

Once your blood has carried alcohol up into the brain it immediately has an impact on multiple circuits and numerous neurons, the key impact being that it triggers a flood of dopamine, that lovely chemical associated with pleasure. Dopamine makes us feel good. This is basically the reason why we drink. However, according to Grisel it's problematic if we rely on a dopamine-producing substance like alcohol to make us feel good, because doing so means we're relying on an area of the brain (the mesolimbic pathway, in case you're interested) that conveys a transient good time and not a stable sense of well-being. This is, she says, because dopamine, as good as it makes us feel, fundamentally signals only the eager anticipation of pleasure, and not the deep sort of pleasure derived from actual satisfaction or contentment.[3]

Alcohol also sparks dopamine in another circuit of the brain, the nigrostriatal pathway, and this is the area that enables us to move towards or away from something stimulating. In the case of a drug like alcohol, we're encouraged by the nigrostriatal pathway to move towards it. So not only is alcohol hitting the mesolimbic pathway, giving us lip-smacking excitement, but also it hits the nigrostriatal pathway, encouraging us to move towards it.[4] The dual messages we're receiving from deep within our brain's reward pathways are 'I like it' and 'I want it'. It's a double whammy.

There's so much more that goes on inside our heads in relation to alcohol (I am summarising massively here), but the other thing that should be noted is that the brain doesn't simply take alcohol in and keep on acting on it as it's forced to (by releasing dopamine, et cetera)—over time the brain reshapes itself to compensate. This is the whole 'building up a tolerance' thing. It happens because the brain decides that the constant flood of dopamine it's being forced to push out is too great, so it begins to downregulate (suppress its response). The dopamine receptors thin out so that they don't respond as enthusiastically.[5] This leads us to need more of the drug to get the same effect. And, because your dopamine receptors are thin, when alcohol is not present your natural dopamine levels drop below the average resting point, leaving you feeling bleak. Hence why people often feel low and miserable the day after a drinking session, or on non-drinking days, and why they feel the need for a drink to pick themselves up again.

The reason I'm putting all these pointy-headed facts in is to break it down and show that the way we feel when drinking isn't mysterious; it makes perfect scientific sense. The good news is that, just as dopamine receptors can downregulate if they're overused, they can also regenerate when they stop being pounded quite so much. Which is why, eight years after quitting, I no longer feel the need for wine to improve my day. Isn't the brain a clever thing?

Alcohol is classed as a depressant, not so much because of the downregulating impact it has on our dopamine receptors, but because it slows down the central nervous system—brain activity and body functioning—making us feel relaxed, less inhibited and sleepier. (The other classes of drugs are stimulants, like caffeine and cocaine, which speed up the brain and body, making us more alert and energetic, and hallucinogens, like LSD or magic mushrooms, which alter what we experience through our senses.[6]) People are often surprised when they find out that alcohol is a depressant because it feels like a 'pick-me-up' drug. And yeah, it can have that effect for the first couple of drinks, because small amounts of alcohol affect areas of the brain that make us chattier and more animated. However the true, depressive impacts of booze swiftly come in after the first few drinks. Things like slurred speech, muddled thinking, slow reactions, stumbling, double vision, hazy memories—all obvious signs that someone's a few sheets to the wind.

From a purely female perspective there are a few additional sciency-type points to make about alcohol. Firstly, if a woman and a man drink the same amount, the woman's blood alcohol will almost always be higher. This is because we generally have a higher proportion of body fat (and therefore less body water) than men. Alcohol is held in body water, so the alcohol held in women is more concentrated.[7] Another reason why alcohol impacts females more is because we produce smaller quantities of the enzyme in the liver called alcohol dehydrogenase, which helps to break down alcohol.[8] Our hormones also play a part, particularly as we age and go through menopause. Our body composition changes, and the likelihood of experiencing stress and depression during that massive life change has been proven to trigger the onset of alcohol abuse or worsen established alcohol misuse.[9] Many women say alcohol makes hot flashes and night sweats worse (some studies have found this to be the case, others haven't, so the scientific jury is out on this one). Oh, and there's also apparently solid evidence to show that women's brains are more sensitive to alcohol than men's are, and that many of the behavioural aspects of alcoholism progress more rapidly among women than among men.[10] So yeah, sorry, ladies. The news for us isn't good. As Dr Lars Møller, Programme Manager, Alcohol and Illicit Drugs at the World Health Organization, puts it, 'Alcohol is quite simply more damaging to women.'[11]

10.

Mary

'This is going to make my body go limp.
It's going to take away my pain.'

I was brought up as Exclusive Brethren and drinking was taboo, so I kinda grew up with unhealthy beliefs about it. I did get drunk when I was about eighteen months old with communion wine. It was a big joke in our family, but who knows what it did to my brain? The only time when I really did enjoy just a casual glass of wine or something like that was out at a dinner, and that was quite functional.

I moved away when I was eighteen to start training as a nurse and that was more of a party environment. If I did go out and my glass was empty, there was the pressure to drink more. I used to have to pretend that my glass had just been topped up, and keep it at a level so that I didn't get more and more pissed. I remember getting gut aches on gin and tonic, going into the bathroom and my tummy just absolutely griping from having drunk too much. So it wasn't a healthy pattern for me. It was always either full-on or 'I'm backing off and can't touch this stuff any more for a while.'

Then I had a terrible back injury and had a spinal fusion. Shortly after that my mother died so I moved back home. Then in the space of just a few years I also lost my father, my nana, my grandad, my auntie, my uncle and then another uncle. Seven deaths in a short space of time. I was just so vulnerable and weak and desperate, really. An absolute mess. So I started self-medicating and drinking quite a lot.

By the time I met my husband I had healed a bit. We got married and had a son. I didn't drink during my pregnancy, didn't even have coffee. The catalyst for me going back to drinking was not being able to manage the ongoing back pain, and I was getting a lot of pressure from the church we were attending to perform and play the piano, and I couldn't say no. Then two friends died and the trigger of the grief—it all just became too much. That's when I went back to booze. I had all this unresolved emotional pain and drink at least relieved it a little bit.

In the evenings after I'd worked hard all day and I'd fed my husband and my son I'd think, *This is my reward. This will relax me. This is going to make my body go limp. It's going to take away my pain.* But what I didn't know was that it was creeping up and I was getting obnoxious, saying awful things. It got so bad, it nearly destroyed my marriage.

I got a really big fright from my husband, who is quite calm normally. He was getting so upset at my drinking and some of the things I was saying when drunk, and he knew that we needed help. He got so frustrated one night he actually put his hand through the wall. That was a real wake-up call for me. I was like, *Woah, he's really pissed off with this behaviour*. I'm glad I had a brave husband who didn't hit me and hit the wall instead. But even with his outburst I wasn't quite ready to accept that I had to stop, so the drinking still went on, very subtly. I got a little bit sneaky because he was like, 'We're not having any in the house.'

We moved way out into the country where you couldn't get alcohol, so it became like a natural detox without me really trying to do it. But I was in a real game with it. I was in a cycle of, *I'm going to have some, but I don't really need this, but yes I do, but no I don't*. I'd decide to have some alcohol but then I'd feel really guilty. I didn't bring booze home, but sometimes when I was getting the groceries, or if I was in a lot of pain with my back, I'd sneak out so that my husband wouldn't see it and grab some cheapo cask wine in town. I'd sit in the park to drink it and just breathe. I felt like the alcohol was making my body relax, and easing the pain. It was something just for me, something that was just mine. That went on for a while and it was going okay until I blew it out at a wedding.

We'd driven for an hour and a half to get to this wedding, and my back was in a lot of pain from sitting in the car for that long. Once we arrived I just started knocking back the free wine. They didn't have any substantial food there; it was just finger bits. My sister must have recognised I was getting plastered because I do remember her saying, 'You should be alternating that wine with water', so things were going downhill a bit then. I remember putting some shoes on to go back to the car with my niece, then my memory gets a bit patchy. All of a sudden I'm sobbing into a cup at a coffee shop. I don't even remember how I got there. I was wailing, 'Where's my son? Is somebody looking after my son?' Then I completely lost it and vomited into the cup, and then apparently vomited four times in the back of the car. My sister-in-law had to shower me. I woke up to my darling brother sitting on the bed saying, 'I think you better go teetotal.' I didn't even know where my son was; he'd been pretty affected by my behaviour. That's a rock bottom.

After I came home I rang AA, and I got a guy called John. I said, 'Do you think I've got a drinking problem?'—still trying to deny it! And he said, 'The very fact that you've rung me, my dear friend, is an indication that yes, you probably have.' That was it, I reached a point within. I fell on my knees and asked God to help and I believe it was Him who gave me the power to stop.

As I started recovering, the stories started coming out. My husband and my son told me how revolting I became when I drank. My son said to me, 'You know, Mum, you really said some awful things.' I had to ask them to forgive me. I remember hugging my husband and saying 'I'm so sorry, I had no idea.' I took myself off to a psychiatrist who helped me work on things, particularly all the grief I'd experienced in my life.

You don't actually realise alcohol is making the problem worse until you stop it. Then you're left with this kind of, *Well, what am I going to do now? How am I going to deal with this?* It was about asking myself, *What works for me to make me breathe and calm down?* For me now it's a prayer, nice music, a walk in the garden or on the beach. I put my feet on the ground and touch the earth and lift my face to the sun, and it's just glorious.

I've also accepted that life isn't glorious all the time. I needed to realise things like this before, without adding the depressant into the mix. Because I've since realised that booze actually escalated the problem and added to it, made me more depressed. It wasn't until I stopped that I realised—you can't do it when you've got alcohol in your life because you're just a bit foggy.

In the six years since I got sober I've learned so much about myself. I was a yes person; my default was always to say 'yes' because I loved helping people. I was a nurse. That was my whole script. I married a 'no' person, and in sixteen years we've balanced each other out with that. I've learned there's a nice healthy balance somewhere in the middle there. Women are capable of doing everything, but I think we forget that we actually do have a physical body and that we do have a timeframe—just 24 hours a day—and we can't possibly do it all in one day. Sometimes we get a bit manic and think we can do the entire lot, and we miss out on self-care and self-nurturing. We put ourselves last.

I still have the terrible back pain. It's hard when I go out somewhere, because sitting for long periods of time gives my back a bit of grief. Sometimes I take painkillers, but where before I just used to swallow them down willy-nilly with booze, now I'm in charge and don't take them unless I really need to. People can't understand: they look at me and I'm slim, I look completely healthy, so they have absolutely no idea what pain I have to manage. At our home in the evenings what I do is I say, 'Hey, guys, I'm getting to that full-time feeling,' and I just go and lie down on the couch. I just go and lie down horizontally, because that relieves the pain in my back from the fusion. Problem solved.

With emotional stuff, I've learned to just take some time out, go for a walk outside in nature, get in the bath, hug my husband. A decent hug is very soothing, a huge relief. And my son still does it, even though he's a teenager! Hugs are very important in our family. What I was doing in drinking all that booze was actually putting a wall between me and them and pushing them away. Making them part of the problem when actually they were part of my answer.

11.

Disconnection

Sometimes I'm right back there. Slumped on the sofa, TV on, eyes glazed, glass in hand. The scent of cheap red wine wafts up as I bend my elbow and take a big slurp. There's a definite wobble in my hand. What is this? Glass number four? Five? I slurp again, draining the glass, then lurch up and stumble my way to the kitchen. I make two pieces of toast, then two more, slathering each one with copious amounts of butter. I top up my glass once more before stumbling back to the sofa to flop down again. Is it the Kardashians I'm watching? Who cares. I'm disconnected from the tele, I'm disconnected from the room, I'm disconnected from myself. I'm a numb, dulled, sozzled woman, full of wine and toast and blurry thoughts. If I cut myself right now I'd hardly feel it. If I watched something heartfelt, I'd hardly register it. If I was having a conversation, I'd barely be in it. I am the opposite of grounded and present. I am barely there. Just a sad, soaked, disconnected version of myself.

If I look back over all my years of heavy drinking, this is

the image that sticks in my mind, the bit that distresses me the most. It's not all the money I pissed away, or the nights I lost to hazy memory. It's not the sloppy behaviour that others may have judged me for or the bad decisions that made me unsafe. No, it's the fact that night after night after night (the most notable thing about my drinking habit was that I rarely took a day off) I slurped wine, and in the process dulled and disconnected myself. I didn't realise it then, but I can see it clearly now. The biggest impact of my drinking on me was disconnection. And I'm not alone in that.

Over the past five years at livingsober.org.nz I've been publishing weekly in-depth stories from people in long-term recovery. There are currently over 150 of these Sober Stories sitting on our site, all powerful, moving and unique, but I can say without a shadow of a doubt that the one thing that unites them is talk of disconnection. 'I felt numb and disconnected,' admits Sue in her story. 'I felt disconnected from the world and those around me,' Liv tells me in hers. 'Being without my best buddy, alcohol, revealed to me the extent of my disconnection with the world,' shares Alison.

Crystal McLean has worked as a counsellor for many years, predominantly with women who are struggling with their drinking. 'What I've observed is they lose the ability to actually get in touch with who they are,' she tells me over the phone from Auckland. 'They part from themselves, their soul. It's like they're stunted. They don't know how to express how they feel, they don't know how to express their emotions, because they've used alcohol to suppress all of those things. I see them as being encased in this metal pod where they don't even know who they are anymore. That's usually when people start reaching out. It might be causing problems in their relationship or with their children, but usually the first person that it's impacted on is themselves. They lose who they are.'

Neuroscientist Judith Grisel calls alcohol 'a neurological sledgehammer' because of the way it affects virtually all aspects of neural functioning. 'One or two drinks help to blur the edges, and a reduction in anxiety promotes relaxation,' she says in *Never Enough: The neuroscience and experience of addiction*. But, beyond one or two drinks, relaxation quickly turns sour: 'As the concentration in the blood and brain increases, judgment is impaired and motor skills decline while risky behaviour increases, along with memory and concentration problems, emotional volatility, loss of coordination, including slurred speech, and confusion.'[1] Stumbling, slurring and not knowing what you're watching on TV are signs of alcohol intoxication, but what about the hidden, internal impacts of letting this sledgehammer loose in our brains? Things like failing to register how we're truly feeling about something, not being able to properly process our emotional responses to things, not hearing what other people are trying to tell us or failing to empathise with others' experiences. These are the powerful, vital functions our brains are constantly performing, the things that make us humans not robots, the things that connect us to ourselves and to everyone around us. They're hard to do when our neural functions are being slowed, our judgement is impaired, we're struggling with memory and concentration problems and suffering from emotional volatility and confusion. Simply put, alcohol disconnects us from the sharp edges of human experience.

You might want to be disconnected from the sharp edges

of human experience if, say, you need a limb amputated and there's no anaesthetic around, like I saw them do once on *The Walking Dead* when a character got bitten by a zombie and they had to cut off his arm before he turned into a zombie himself and there were no proper drugs around so they gave him a bottle of whisky and he gulped big mouthfuls of it in between screams. That sort of human experience might be a good one to accompany with booze. But, if you're an ordinary person trying to live a rich, full life, it's possibly not such a great idea.

It wasn't for me. I spent so many hours under the influence of alcohol, dulled and numb and disconnected, I never gave myself much time to clearly think and feel. Add in all the hours I spent planning my drinking, wrestling with myself about whether to drink or not, recovering from drinking and feeling bad about drinking, and it's no surprise that I found myself sober at 40, not really knowing who I was. How could I possibly? I never gave myself any good stretches of time to think things through or process stuff. I never gave myself a chance to pause and reflect, to truly understand myself. What made me feel good, what made me feel bad, how could I self-soothe, how could I lift myself up, how did I feel about my parents' divorce or that boyfriend who once taunted me with a loaded gun? All I did was glug, glug, glug, creating noise, distraction and disconnection.

'But what if I don't want to feel the sadness of my awful marriage break-up?' I hear you cry. 'What if I don't want to feel the grief of losing my mum or the stress of dealing with a boss who's a narcissistic bully?' It's understandable to want to numb those things away. The problem is, if we try to numb and disconnect from one thing, we numb and disconnect from everything—good and bad. Alcohol is a neurological sledgehammer, remember? It dulls it all. Research professor Brené Brown explains it this way in her famous TED Talk 'The power of vulnerability': 'You cannot selectively numb emotion. You can't say, here's the bad stuff. Here's vulnerability, here's grief, here's shame, here's fear, here's disappointment, I don't want to feel these. When we numb those, we numb joy, we numb gratitude, we numb happiness.'[2] Numb the bad and you numb the good. Drink all the time and you end up disconnected. And that's a real bummer. 'Connection is why we're here,' states Brown in her talk, which you really should watch if you haven't already. 'It's what gives purpose and meaning to our lives. This is what it's all about.'

12.

Belinda

'I said to my therapist recently,
"I just don't feel like I feel anything."'

I grew up in beautiful Cape Town. It's a bit of a badge of honour to be a big drinker in South Africa. My mom didn't drink very much, but my dad was quite a big drinker. He'd come home and have a couple of bottles of beer every evening, and he always enjoyed a party. His father, my grandfather, had a very successful career, but he was a high-functioning alcoholic and would drink a bottle of gin across the course of the day. It wasn't fun for my dad, and I think it's left him really emotionally crippled.

We sometimes had wine as children around the table, but only tiny little glasses. I probably seriously got into it when I was fourteen or fifteen. I drank every weekend all the way through my teens. We'd go and buy bottles of terrible, cheap, sweet wine and then head to the school discos. Once

I left school at eighteen I moved to the UK to do my OE, and I've never moved home again.

When I first got to the UK, drinking during the week wasn't a big priority, and I would only buy one bottle of wine for the week. Weekends, however, were spent down at the pub and out late dancing in the clubs. As I've ended up with more money I've been able to drink a lot more. In my late twenties I got a boyfriend who drank a lot and we started drinking a bottle of wine every night—that was when it started to get much more serious. Whenever I had a day off from work the next day I would always take the opportunity to go out on the town and get shit-faced, because I could and it was fun. But I've also gone to work very hungover many times over the years. I've been hungover every weekend as an adult since I could afford it. In all fairness, so were all my mates. The thing that always struck me was that really I didn't want to be hungover every weekend, but Friday would come around again, and I could never say no to the drink.

Once I've had two or three glasses, I'm suddenly like, *Wahay, more is obviously better! We're only going to have more fun! Woo-hoo!* I know people who go, 'Oh I've got a nice buzz, so I'll just maintain this nice buzz,' and they can have a water, and then they can have maybe a mocktail, and then another glass of wine. I've never been able to do this. For me the drinking just escalates over the course of the evening. I've never left the restaurant with a drink still there. My husband will get up to go pay and I'm like, 'Where are we going? There's wine left!'

I've been having an ongoing dialogue with myself about my alcohol use for many years. When I think back to some of the more hectic things that have happened in my life, I've certainly gone straight to alcohol as a kind of numbing device, to take the edge off. What's been the alarm for me is being so hungover that I'm cancelling stuff because I feel so ill—when I can't get out of bed on a Saturday morning to go to a brunch with my mates because I feel like shit. And it's not just once; it's almost every weekend that something will get cancelled.

After I moved to New Zealand I came across a website that had all these new 'drink aware' tools. How much is a standard drink? How do you test whether you're a problem drinker? It got me thinking. I don't think I'm an alcoholic but I do think that I've probably got a bit of a, well, I don't know. I don't know how you would classify it. Ever since then I've tried to have alcohol-free days each week, but I've always struggled with it. I just find it so easy to go, *One doesn't hurt*, or, *Tomorrow can be the alcohol-free day*. I go through phases when I can't remember having an alcohol-free day, unless I have a stonking hangover. But even then I'd consider hair of the dog.

When I got pregnant with my little boy, who is now three and a half, I was slightly worried about it. I wondered how the not drinking was going to go while I was pregnant. Genuinely, I was like, *How's this actually gonna pan out? Am I going to be able to do this?* Thankfully I just didn't feel like alcohol. I did drink a little while I was breastfeeding, which was for the most part of a year, but it was rubbish. I'd have one glass of wine and I would feel so hungover the next day. It was so disappointing. The struggle for me was about trying to have fun without booze. Normally if I go out I'll have a glass of wine before I go, a glass of wine before dinner, a glass of wine with dinner. But when I was breastfeeding I just felt like rubbish the next day after drinking. So there was a constant kind of annoyance, like, *If I can't have wine what's the point?* I really struggled with that. It was this feeling that if I didn't have the alcohol, I was missing out on the next level of fun or the next level of connection. Which is rubbish, but it's just such a strong feeling I had. It's only now that I can really properly drink again, three and a half years on. I went out to a party recently and it was like, *Whoa, cool. Yay, I'm back.*

I've done quite a lot of therapy work over my life. Sometimes for specific traumatic incidents that have happened, at other times just if I'm struggling. I find it really beneficial. I said to my therapist recently, 'I just don't feel like I feel anything.' I've felt totally disconnected and numb for years. I remember on my wedding day thinking, *This is nice, but why am I not excited? This is meant to be the happiest day of my life.* There was no joy. So I'm doing all this work with my therapist at the moment, and some really interesting stuff has come out around my childhood. In a nutshell, I had two parents who looked after me, educated me and provided for me, but in their own different ways were simply not present. Neither took (or takes) any true interest in my life. My dad was off in his own world, and my mum was just a bit self-absorbed, and when it came down to it didn't really want children. This has resulted in a very complex relationship with my mother.

I used to talk to Mum about stuff and I just don't anymore. I don't let her in. I don't tell her anything because she just shits all over it. She doesn't even realise she is doing it. This has been happening since forever. There's no space for me and I don't think there ever has been.

Lately I've experienced a white-hot anger that I haven't experienced before. It feels like a complete lack of control. There's a suppressed rage there and I don't know how to cope with it. Sometimes I take it out on my family. I shout a lot. That's partly what's got me seeking help with a therapist right now. In the past couple of weeks something came up with her. There was this whole 'sense of self' moment that we had. She said to me, 'You've got to realise that you've put up a lot of walls and a lot of barriers because of all the stuff that you've been through.' And I was like, 'That's not good. How do I get rid of those? How do I become myself? How do I become more open?' She said, 'That's a good thing. Don't underestimate why nature does these things. And don't knock yourself about for the fact that that's happened. But give yourself permission to be yourself when you feel you can.' It was such an enlightening moment and that feeling stayed with me for the whole weekend and into the following week. And I didn't drink for the whole week. I went back to her the following week and it was the first time I talked to her about alcohol. I was like, 'I've always had this really complex fight with alcohol, which for some reason I've never thought to mention to you before. But this last week I've not felt the need to drink.' After the session my husband said, 'You could not drink tonight.' I said, 'Steady on, that's a bit extreme. I'm not here to prove anything.'

I don't want to give up alcohol completely. I just wish I was more in control of how I enjoy it. Wrestling with it is so tiring. The constant, *Should I or shouldn't I? Have I taken enough bottles to the party? Should I have another drink?* All that wasted energy. So I'm not all in, but I'm open to it. My therapist says it's brave to do all the work I'm doing on myself but I feel like I'm just curious. There's something going on, so let's sort it out. There's no excitement in life but there's also no extreme sadness. I want to start feeling joy. I want to start feeling again.

13.

Vulnerability

I sat down to write this chapter like I do all my chapters: with a rough idea of what I wanted to say but no clear idea of how I was going to say it. Normally, this goes perfectly well for me and over the course of many hours' writing the idea grows and the chapter takes shape. But with this one that's not how it went. With this one I struggled right from the get-go. Just a few lines in and I got stuck trying to make my point without sounding like an arsehole. How could I talk about drinking making women vulnerable without making it sound like I think they're to blame if something bad happens to them? Around and around I went, typing sentences then deleting them, at a loss about how to raise the issue without making anyone feel bad. It was a hellishly difficult thing to do, almost impossible, I thought, to the point where I contemplated ditching the chapter altogether. Until one day I had a genius idea: 'I need Steph.'

Steph Anderson is a totally awesome addiction nurse with years of experience helping women turn their lives around.

She's smart, warm, wise, amazingly grounded and hugely devoted to her work. I first met her at a conference four years ago, and we've kept in touch ever since. The instant she came to my mind while struggling with this chapter, I knew she was the perfect person to help get it out. So I made contact, explained my predicament and we scheduled a phone call. The resulting conversation is what you're about to read below.

Me: I need your help.

Steph Anderson: What's up?

Me: I'm writing about all of the different ways alcohol can impact on women's lives, and I want to write about vulnerability and safety—how when you drink past a certain point you're vulnerable to bad things happening to you.

Steph: Okay.

Me: But I don't know how to do this without it sounding like I'm suggesting that women are to blame somehow if something bad happens to them while they're under the influence. Because the only person who is to blame if there's any sort of violence or sexual assault is the person who did it, right?

Steph: Right. If a rape happens or a sexual assault or any type of violence, then the perpetrator is entirely to blame.

Me: But there are issues around vulnerability and safety for women when they're drinking—how can I talk about that and not make it about blame?

Steph: Hmmm, it is a bit of a minefield that one, but we do need to have some brave discussions around this because many women's lives are affected in this way.

Me: So let's have a discussion then. But first, remind me about your experience and expertise in this area.

Steph: I'm an addiction nurse specialist, and I've been working in this field for 25 years.

Me: And you've dealt with thousands of women in that time?

Steph: Oh yeah, thousands. Thousands and thousands of women.

Me: Have you often had discussions about bad things that have happened to women where alcohol was involved?

Steph: Many times. Once I've built a space where women can be honest, feel respected and able to talk about stuff freely, I say, 'You know, it's really common when you've been drinking that you make bad choices. Have you ever made any bad choices that still play on your mind or still affect how you function in the world now?' Without fail the majority of women will say 'yes', they have put themselves in positions where they have been very vulnerable, or been assaulted, or made bad choices or continued bad choices, that sort of stuff. It's very, very, very common.

Me: Are they carrying guilt and shame around that?

Steph: Absolutely. When I think about my career in the world of substance use problems and all the women I've dealt with, that is the overwhelming feature that stands out: women feel guilty about losing control and letting stuff happen. They move very quickly from 'This person did this to me' to 'I lost control' or 'I let that happen'. And that adds to their trauma massively. They feel bad about it and feel they can't talk to people about it.

Me: Is part of the problem that they're judged by outsiders when things happen to them while they're under the influence?

Steph: For sure. How women are treated in courts is still pretty appalling at times. If a woman has been raped and she was intoxicated when she was raped, she's still much more likely not to be believed.

Me: There are so many court cases concerning sexual assault and rape where the defence focus on the intoxication level of the victim.

Steph: I imagine the true amount of sexual assault is massively underreported because women don't feel that they are ever going to be believed, or they actually feel responsible themselves because they got pissed and it happened.

Me: What about the judgement they might receive from professionals like emergency services and others?

Steph: Over the years I've had a huge amount of trouble getting women with substance use issues who've been assaulted or sexually attacked into crisis housing or support services, because they have a big issue with women who use alcohol. There's a judgement attached to it. It also happens an awful lot with ambulance officers, the police, nurses and doctors in emergency departments. If you've been assaulted they might be dismissive of you because you smell of alcohol. If that's your first interaction with a professional, then the blame is already embedded, the guilt starts to grow, and then you're less likely to seek help for yourself, aren't you?

Me: So what would you say to a woman who's been in that position where they've been drunk, something's happened, they've felt judged and then they blame themselves? What do you want to say to them?

Steph: I would be saying to them that this is an experience that they need to think about. And that they need some help to understand the mechanism of it in order to change how they feel about it and to prevent it happening again.

Me: And also, you're not to blame for this.

Steph: No. But it's a balance, isn't it, because you don't want women going out saying to themselves, 'Oh, well, if I get drunk and shit happens, it's not my fault.'

Me: Yeah, okay. Gosh, it's complex, isn't it?

Steph: It's a minefield.

Me: So putting the judgement thing aside, how do you, in your treatment and care of women, address the fact that when they drank they potentially made themselves vulnerable?

Steph: I say, 'This happens to a lot of women, but you are not to blame. You never set out having that drink at the beginning of the night thinking, *I'm going to be raped or beaten later.* Did you? You never intended for this to happen.' And I emphasise to them that after a certain point they're not in control. 'Your thinking brain, your rational brain, got totally hijacked by alcohol and you were not yourself.' One of the most powerful things to say to women is, 'You were not yourself. This is not the real you.'

Me: I like that: 'Your rational brain got totally hijacked by alcohol.' So there's a separation there. Yes, it was you who was drinking and these things happened. But you weren't yourself, you weren't your rational self, you're not to blame, that shouldn't have happened to you. And then kind of moving forward from that position of strength.

Steph: There's a very powerful visual thing that I do with women. Basically it's an axis where on the left-hand side you have power, and along the bottom axis you have an amount of drinks. On the left axis, you start with two dots. One is the rational brain and the other is The Beast, which is what we call the drinking brain. When you start at one drink, your rational brain is still at the top of the left-hand axis. The drinking brain—The Beast—creeps up a little bit. Then you have another drink and the rational brain moves down a little and The Beast moves up. And then you just carry on that progression. The more drinks you have, the more that the power of the rational brain declines and the power of The Beast increases, and there's a crossover point. I would say to women, 'At that crossover point, you no longer have control.'

Me: That visualisation is powerful.

Steph: Oh, it is. And we all know that there's a crossover point at which we no longer have control, because that's why we have laws about not drink driving or handling heavy machinery and such things. We know how alcohol affects our ability to judge and coordinate. The key is to get people to identify where the crossover is for them. It might be two drinks. For some people it's the first drink. I say to women, 'Where did the horrible stuff happen?' And when they say it happened at this point of the bottom axis, I tell them, 'There's no way that you could be in control. It's biological—you weren't able to make any good decisions.'

Me: I like that thing about creating a separation from the things that happened when you were under the influence. So you can go, 'Yes, it was me but I was drinking and I wasn't myself.' Can you talk about that again, because I really think that's powerful in terms of shifting the guilt and shame.

Steph: It's so powerful. The Beast is a way of conceptualising when it's not the real you, because that's when your primitive, drinking brain is in control. It's driven by alcohol. That's the most powerful thing: starting to figure out when you're not really there and It is there. Calling it 'It'.

Me: Yeah, we use names like 'The Wine Witch' or, my personal favourite, 'The Inner Booze-Pig'.

Steph: I think about the times when I've been drunk and I haven't been myself, it's not the real me. It's something else. So I think that's the biggest thing to say to women: 'This isn't the real you. The real you is still there but it's being plastered over by alcohol.'

Me: So if we know there's that point in the night when the rational brain has clocked off, how do you work with women to figure out what's best for them in terms of alcohol?

Steph: Well, I think it is about helping them figure it out for themselves. Giving them the tools to figure it out and using the techniques that a skilled practitioner has. Getting them to the point where the crossover point becomes much clearer in their mind.

Me: Have you found in your work over the years that it takes a lot for women to get over any self-blame they may have for things that have happened?

Steph: Yes. Because there's no doubt about it, the consequences for women who drink are far greater than for men. I see it time and time again.

Me: How important is it for women, do you think, to not make themselves vulnerable? To be in the best place they can to deal with things when they happen, whether it be an abusive boyfriend or a predatory guy in the bar. How important is it that women aren't compromised in those sorts of scenarios so that they can be their best selves, making their best decisions?

Steph: I think it's absolutely vital because, as we know, women keep our society together, they keep families together, and they raise our youngsters. But there's also perhaps a deeper thing to think about, which is for some women, what's gone wrong in the past? We know that there's a huge percentage of underlying or coexisting mental-health issues or trauma-based stuff already in play. And if women have had shit lives, have had sexual abuse as a child or whatever, then they're more likely to turn to drink. And then they're more likely to put themselves in positions where that abuse is perpetuated. There's a bigger cycle at play for a lot of women.

Me: That's right, and I am going to talk about that later in the book (see Part Four) when I talk about possible causes for women relying heavily on alcohol. But for now, in terms of this vulnerability issue, you're saying the best thing is to be honest with yourself and be mindful of where your crossover point is with drinking. The world, unfortunately, is not always a safe place for women, so it's important we give ourselves the best chance we can of keeping safe.

Steph: Yes. And, if something bad has happened in your life, try to get some support from an outside perspective. Find the strength to acknowledge to yourself what's happened as a result of your drinking, and find someone else who you can talk to honestly about that. That's part of the process of trying to rebuild self-esteem. Because we know that, when people drink or use drugs, often their underlying value system goes astray. They do things that they would never normally do, or they allow people to do things to them that they would never normally allow. So it's about realigning your moral compass. If you don't do that, if you don't solidify your values, and your beliefs about yourself as a person who has the ability to say no, look after yourself and stand up for other people, then you sort of continue to drift through and you have your self-esteem drop and you can still be a very vulnerable person.

Me: Okay, well I feel we've just scratched the surface of this issue but hopefully it will get people thinking, and if need be feeling empowered to go talk to someone and get help from an outside perspective. Thank you so much, Steph.

Steph: Happy to help.

14.

Pamela

'He said, "I will fucking kill
you"—and meant it.'

I have effectively a teetotal mother, and a father who
every time he drank got the hiccups. There was never
any anger from him or violence. Never anything, just the
hiccups. He died of a heart attack when I was fourteen. It
was so traumatic because it was literally overnight. Mum
didn't cope at all. Right before my fifteenth birthday, I got
absolutely annihilated at a party and lost my virginity. It
was the first time I ever got drunk. It wasn't a happy thing.
I wouldn't say that it wasn't consensual; I just had no idea
of what it was. Like, none. I knew about the birds and the
bees, but I didn't know the tangibles. So in terms of informed
consent, none whatsoever.

I got rebellious after that, and I used to leave the house
in the middle of the night to go nightclubbing. I really could

have done with a parent who was around, but Mum had completely flaked out. I was fortunate that I had a good group of friends who kept an eye on me. We drank, but not that much, and because we were always dancing we always exercised it off. After school finished I moved away to study. There was some heavy drinking that went on there but I didn't like the masculinity associated with it, so I ended up leaving after nine months and moving back home to continue on in the dance-party scene. I moved over to London for a while, then I came back to NZ and that's when I met Jon.

Jon was a child of alcoholics, a child of excess. He either drank until he passed out, or he didn't touch it. There was no middle ground. When I was with him, we drank, and the more time we spent together, the more excessive it became. Huge amounts. I went along with it because I can drink quite happily. At first it was nice; he anchored me. He adored me, and I absolutely adored him, it was a really deep connection. We were really compatible, had a good time together and created great stuff together. Like really cool stuff: cool music, cool arts, cool performance, cool stuff.

We moved to a big city in Asia where we used to throw dance parties. He was in a band and I would do all of the technical stuff and performance-art installations. I also got a good job working in a university, earning great money for not many hours a week. Life was good, life was easy. It was a crazy, 24/7, constant, moving, creative, exciting environment. It was all on and we used alcohol as sugar to keep us going. We'd have all-night parties, get home at dawn, put on music, chill, relax, continue on and party. The relationship was generally good, but in hindsight it wasn't healthy because he was very controlling and would often put me down. But at the time I was oblivious. It was very hard to be aware of what was going on in that crazy, busy, boozy environment. But there were alarm bells. One Christmas Jon ended up comatose under a table, literally in the foetal position. I remember thinking, *That's really not healthy.*

We started working with the local government, getting huge grants to put on festivals and parties. That's when the wheels started falling off. After we'd done one big festival, drinking tons, Jon actually had a complete and utter meltdown. He lost his shit—it was so extreme, so explosive. We got through that fight okay, but the relationship slowly turned very bad. His behaviour deteriorated and he got more violent and more aggressive towards me. He was always drinking when this would happen, and I would be as well. We'd have drunken fights and he'd get physical. It was extreme, it was heightened, it was intense, it was charged. I was in fight-or-flight mode all the time. I had a little inner dialogue telling me *This isn't right* to a certain degree, but I always thought that I could fix it.

We had a child together, and once that happened it became very clear to me that I had two children. Real issues started emerging. Jon got very jealous of our baby and the attention I was giving him. He literally said to me one day, 'What we could do is put the baby up for adoption, and then we can figure this out.' The violence got really bad. We started going to counselling, and after our second counselling session we went out drinking afterwards. The baby was at home with the nanny. While we were out in the bar I did something that made Jon mad, and he just lost it. Completely lost it. I left him at the bar and went home to relieve the nanny. He followed me home and beat the shit out of me. I'd never before seen somebody turn animalistic, threaten to kill and actually look like they mean it. It was literally like a shutter went down over his eyes and he said, 'I will fucking kill you'—and meant it. He ripped hair out of my head, I had blood pouring out, then he kicked me out onto the street. I ended up going into hospital overnight and had to walk home the next day covered with bloodstains, bruising, bandages. I didn't leave straight away, but the situation got worse—he no longer needed the alcohol to get violent. Then he started hitting our child and that was it. We left him.

I came home and slept on my mum's couch for two years. I'd been drinking heavily through the end of the relationship, and when I got home I drank like a fish, one or two bottles of wine a night, hiding the empties. But I slowly managed to get myself together. It's nearly ten years on now and I've got a good job, bought my own apartment and have stopped the heavy drinking. I don't usually drink more than two glasses at a time. Maybe once or twice a year I drink two bottles in a sitting. I made the quick realisation that if I drink too much wine at night I don't sleep. And in order to be able to do my job I need to sleep. So I've managed to rein it right back. But I do have an ongoing relationship with alcohol. I know the people at the bottle store, and they know me. I've never gone longer than three weeks without drinking.

When I do drink more heavily, it's really clearly related to emotional strain. It's clearly related to anything Jon has to do with my life. He's living overseas but is still coming at us. Just a couple of weeks ago I heard he was trying to get at me through the court system, which he's entitled to do even though I've explained the domestic abuse. When I got the call I burst into tears, and I've spent the past two weeks trying to figure out what the hell to do. I don't want to see him. I don't want him seeing me. Everyone's telling me I'm being stalked, so I've had the police here, explaining the situation. But they say there's nothing they can do. I can't get a restraining order because he's not in the country. It's really fucking hard, and it's impacting on my drinking. The last long weekend we just had I drank an entire bottle of vodka.

I would still drink if Jon wasn't around. I like alcohol. I like being educated about it and I like making choices about it, choosing different wines depending on what I'm feeling. I can be like, 'I don't want a pinot. I want a shiraz. Actually, I'm going to drink vodka.' It's quite considered; there's a beauty to it. It gives me a respite, I can intellectualise alcohol as opposed to having to intellectualise shit.

Do you know what fundamentally stops me from drinking too much, too often? It's my child. He's my wake-up call. Because when I'm hungover and tired, I get grumpy and bitchy towards him and that's not fair on him. That's the point when I will beat myself up. He is my rock, my beautiful child who I adore, and the least I can do is give him a stable, loving, considered, safe environment and a mum.

15.

The C words

We can't talk about the impacts of alcohol and not talk about cancer, so here are the facts.

Alcohol causes cancer. Or to put it another way (and apparently this is the same thing): alcohol greatly increases the risk of getting cancer. The strength of evidence on this has led to the World Health Organization classing alcohol as a Group 1 carcinogen—that's the highest level you can get. (Other Group 1 carcinogens are tobacco and arsenic.) Seven different types of cancer have been proven to be caused by alcohol: mouth cancer, pharyngeal (upper throat) cancer, oesophageal (food pipe) cancer, laryngeal (voice box) cancer, breast cancer, bowel cancer and liver cancer. Evidence is also mounting that alcohol increases the risk of melanoma and prostate, lung, stomach and pancreatic cancers.

Not everyone who drinks alcohol will develop cancer, but people who do drink alcohol are more likely to develop cancer than people who don't. No level of alcohol intake is safe in terms of cancer risk, but the more alcohol you drink, the greater your risk of getting cancer. It doesn't seem to make a difference to your cancer risk if you drink alcohol in big binge sessions or steadily throughout the week (and even light drinkers or occasional binge drinkers increase their risk of getting cancer, but by a much smaller amount). All types of alcoholic beverages are risky.

Drinking alcohol has been firmly established as a risk factor for developing breast cancer. Of all the alcohol-related cancers in New Zealand, breast cancer is the most common. Breast cancer is also the leading cause of all alcohol-related deaths among New Zealand women. One standard alcoholic drink a day (around 100 millilitres of wine) leads to a modest increase in breast-cancer risk (5 per cent), and that risk rises by around 10 per cent for every additional standard drink consumed per day. Women who drink 50 grams or more of pure alcohol a day (that's 500 millilitres of wine, or two standard kitchen measuring cups) have a 60 per cent higher risk of getting breast cancer than non-drinkers.[1]

So these are the known, proven, unequivocal facts around alcohol and cancer, and, while they're shocking, what's even more shocking is that many of us are in the dark about it. A 2015 survey published by Cancer Research UK found that public knowledge of alcohol's contribution to cancer was extremely low—only 13 per cent identified cancer as a health condition that could result from drinking. In 2018, none of the participants in a Health Promotion Agency study here in New Zealand and the subsequent report, *Ready to Contemplate? Midlife adults and their relationship with alcohol,* raised any concern about alcohol's link to cancer. Pretty remarkable given the researchers carried out numerous in-depth interviews exploring participants' past and current drinking habits, the things that sometimes trigger them to contemplate change and the things that might be preventing them from changing. The final published report mentioned cancer only once, and then it was only indirectly by someone referring to another family member's health issues.[2]

Even at livingsober.org.nz, where all we do day after day is talk about alcohol and our feelings, cancer rarely gets a mention. I can't actually remember ever hearing one of our community members cite 'not getting cancer' as a reason for quitting drinking. Personally I've never given cancer much thought and almost my whole life has been about alcohol. I never worried about cancer during my twenty-odd years of drinking like a fish, fearing cancer wasn't a motivation in the months I was working hard to get sober, and I rarely think about it eight years on. Maybe a couple of times lately I've had a tiny thought of, *Hopefully I won't get cancer now*, but it's been a fleeting thing, and after researching this chapter I've discovered I'm no less of a candidate than I was when I was drinking. Apparently it can take many years (up to 35 in some cases!) after quitting for your risk level to drop back down to where it was before you started imbibing. That was a joyful discovery. Not.

So why are we not aware of alcohol's links to cancer? Why do we not worry about cancer every time we pour a drink? Why do we not consider cancer risk when evaluating our drinking habits? Why do we not use the fear of cancer to help motivate us to stop? Is it in the 'too hard' basket? Is it too overwhelmingly negative? Is it because talk of 'raising risk levels' is too vague? Is it because we know not everyone who drinks will get cancer so we hope we'll be one of the lucky ones? Professor Jennie Connor, an epidemiologist in the Department of Preventive and Social Medicine at the University of Otago, thinks it's all of the above. 'I think one of the things is that it's quite hard for people to understand intuitively about chronic disease risk. We can say to women, "Every extra drink a day gives you a 10 per cent increase in your breast cancer risk," and they'll go, "Wow, I didn't know that," but they don't change their behaviour because what does that mean? It's sort of technical in a way that it's not very intuitive. It's a slippery idea and it's hard to form an intent to change your behaviour based on a slippery idea.'

I put it to Professor Connor that another reason for us not understanding or accepting alcohol's cancer-causing properties is that the information sits in such stark contrast to the way alcohol is casually presented in our society. 'That's exactly right,' she agrees. 'Marketing is telling us lies. Marketing is telling us it's okay, it's an ordinary product. Just having it sitting on a shelf in the supermarket tells us we're safe to drink it. It reassures people that it's completely normal.'

I'll give you another reason why we don't focus much on alcohol's link to cancer: confirmation bias. That's the other C word the title of this chapter relates to (well, it's a C and a B word together, but . . . you know). According to Wikipedia, confirmation bias is 'the tendency to search for, interpret, favour and recall information in a way that affirms one's prior beliefs or hypotheses'.[3] In other words, we look for and latch on to information that makes us feel good about our drinking. Research linking alcohol to cancer does not make us feel good about our drinking. But reports stating the positive health benefits of alcohol sure do. You've seen the headlines: 'Heart-healthy benefits of red wine'; 'Why red wine could be good for your gut'; 'Drinking wine better than exercise if you want to live a long life'; 'Beer is officially good for you because it reduces heart risk and improves brain health, reveal scientists'; '5 health benefits of drinking a glass of wine every day'. We lap these headlines up, park them in our brains and mentally refer back to them—often. 'It's okay because red wine is good for me,' I told myself time and again as I poured humongous glass after humongous glass of the stuff (red wine was my poison of choice). Confirmation bias in action. Of course, I never thoroughly read any of the reports to find the disclaimers, limitations and caveats showing things were never actually as positive as the headlines made them out to be. Nor did I listen to the many educated voices warning that any potential benefits of alcohol consumption are massively outweighed by the harms. Because none of that would help confirm my bias now, would it?

Another form of confirmation bias is looking for information that points away from alcohol and towards other things as reasons for health issues. That 2018 Health Promotion Agency study I mentioned earlier (which surveyed middle-aged adults about their drinking habits) found that anyone who was suffering negative health impacts that could be associated with or exacerbated by alcohol (like gout or diabetes) were 'quick to seek out or latch onto any information that supports them to continue drinking at higher than recommended levels. An example of this is the explanation a few gave in relation to shellfish or diet being the trigger for their episodes of gout, rather than their alcohol consumption.' That's right—it's the shellfish you ate last night that's causing your tummy upset, not the five bourbon and Cokes you sank. Again, confirmation bias in action. Another way of describing it could be denial.

Speaking of denial, it's worth noting that the biggest problem public-health experts encounter when trying to get the message out about alcohol's links to cancer is the liquor industry. Big Alcohol doesn't want us to know the truth, or, as Professor Connor puts it, 'the industry refuses to acknowledge that alcohol causes cancer', so they work hard at muddying the waters around the facts. They do this in three main ways: by denying the links between alcohol and cancer (either outright denials or denial by selective omission); by distorting the truth (obscuring, misrepresenting or obfuscating the true nature or size of the risk); and by distracting or diverting attention (pointing the finger elsewhere). It's exactly the same tactics the tobacco industry used when they were trying to hide the links between smoking and cancer.

If you want to read more and get really outraged about how the liquor industry is purposely deceiving us about alcohol and cancer, seek out the paper 'How alcohol industry organisations mislead the public about alcohol and cancer'.[4] If reading academic papers ain't your thing, let me just share a couple of lines from their conclusion with you: 'It has often been assumed that, by and large, the alcohol industry, unlike the tobacco industry, has tended not to deny the harms of alcohol. Our analysis shows that, on the contrary, the global alcohol industry is currently actively disseminating misinformation about alcohol and cancer risk, particularly breast cancer.' Yep, you read that right, ladies. They're mostly hiding the truth about the risk to our boobs.

But wait, there's more: 'This study shows that the alcohol industry uses similar tactics to the tobacco industry, to the same ends: to protect its profits to the detriment of public health. The full scale and nature of these activities requires urgent investigation.'[5]

I asked Professor Connor how important is it that people understand the link between cancer and alcohol. 'I think it's important for a number of different reasons,' she told me. 'I think you have a right to know about the health risks associated with any product that's on sale freely. Even if it's age-restricted, you have a right to know what we know about the health risks. If you don't have the information, you don't have the opportunity to make a reasoned decision.

'The other thing is that to not know about the important health effects of alcohol means that people believe it's not essentially harmful. They just believe it's your responsibility to make sure it doesn't harm you—by not drinking too much too often, and so on. If they understood that not all of the problems with alcohol are about the way you drink it, some of them are just inherent in the product itself, that might change the way they see it. If they understand that alcohol is essentially harmful, it might make them less likely to accept the tradition we have of drinking how much and whenever we feel like it.'

16.

Ruth

'I was in my late fifties when I discovered the lumps in my breasts.'

My parents were very cool party people in the 1960s. They were binge drinkers, but it was always at party time, so I began very early to associate good times with alcohol—a legacy we unfortunately passed on to our children. In the seventies, I got into the hippy thing, going down the smoking-dope route. There were kinda clear demarcations back then—you were either a drinker or a pot-smoker or drug-taker. I probably went between the two worlds a bit. I wasn't a big drinker, though, through my teenage years.

My binge drinking really started in the eighties after I'd had children—that was the boozy decade. By then we were moving out of the hippy vibe and more into a heavy-drinking vibe. There was a group of us—three families all with children—living in a big house together in Takapuna [in Auckland]. There was a big group of people flatting next door as well, so there were two big houses. It was fun. We didn't drink every night or anything, but we definitely were the party house. We did things like have netball games in the lounge and dance till we dropped. The Boss screamed from the stereo at 3 a.m., waking both bleary-eyed children and neighbours alike. It was crazy.

I think I knew that it was too much. There were hideous times when you're vomiting and pissing yourself at the same time, thinking, Christ. This is not pretty. But I think there was kind of a freedom and kudos to getting that trashed. Things were changing, we were navigating the whole feminist thing, and it was part of our right to get as trashed as we wanted to. We were exploring, breaking out of the mould of just being mummies and wives, getting in touch with our own wildish natures. We could be those wild women running naked from their house down to the local hotel and swimming in the pool at two in the morning, waking all the neighbours up and running back home again, still naked. Whether we picked up a freedom that men had had to get trashed, or maybe women hadn't given themselves that permission before, I don't know. But I do know we thought that getting trashed was somehow powerful.

By the nineties we'd moved out of that phase and got into women's workshops, counselling and self-improvement. We were all trying to figure ourselves out. We sat in sharing circles, did crazy concerts, drove to hot pools with our bras on the windscreen, lots of naked stuff, lots of sweat lodges and vision quests. It was very liberating. By then I was only drinking alcohol every now and then, because I had four children, including two stepchildren, so I ring-fenced it to not very often. I certainly didn't have to have a drink every day or even every week. Over time, the big binge-drinking sessions became isolated to probably only a few times a year. But I could still do a couple of bottles of chardonnay at lunch. One of the things that curbed my drinking is I just couldn't do the hangovers. It starts to take a toll on your body. It's only later, I guess, that you realise the health risks.

I was in my late fifties when I discovered the lumps in my breasts. I went and got them checked out, and yes, it was cancer. I had a partial mastectomy where they cut out the lumps, and then I had another one because they didn't quite get the margins. I started thinking, *Wow, there's no history of bloody breast cancer in my family*, so I talked to nurses at the hospital asking, 'Why would I get this?' I needed to know something about what caused it so I could try to prevent it recurring. They tried to tell me that I needed to see a counsellor because I was blaming myself. They said, 'We can get you massages, we can provide facials for you, but don't blame yourself. Anyone can get this. It's nothing to do with your lifestyle.' I just did not believe that story. I found it hugely frustrating, actually, the lack of information at that time about the relationship between lifestyle choice and breast cancer. And I very much felt that people did not want me to take responsibility for my breast cancer.

Because I couldn't get any answers out of the medical people, I started doing my own research. Eventually I came to the conclusion that actually a significant amount of the type of cancer I had is to do with lifestyle, including heavy alcohol use, because it is hormone-driven.

So I chose not to have radiotherapy or chemotherapy, and instead changed my lifestyle. I now walk at least every second day, because I found a research paper that said if you walk for 40 minutes four times a week the recurrence of breast cancer is reduced by a huge amount. I try to only drink merlot now, rather than sugar-laden white wine, and only occasionally. And I've changed to a really plant-rich diet. I'm five years clear of cancer, so fingers crossed.

If I'm really stressed nowadays, I'll meditate to get my head in an okay space, to come back to myself and really get a grip on things. Or I'll just talk with a friend. Getting in the sea is also a really big thing. You wouldn't call it exercise—I more bob about—but I'm very happy doing that. All I can do is do everything I can to help myself, and then hopefully not get a recurrence of the cancer. There's no guarantees, I know that. But I am giving myself the best chance and part of that story is not drinking too much alcohol. Hormonally it's not good for us. It just isn't.

I would love to live in a world where we know that we can have fun, and it not be associated with something that's so potentially dangerous. It would be great to live in a world where it wasn't a driver of social events, and where binge drinking, particularly, wasn't so normalised. It destroys families and I see young women so at risk from being so freaking trashed they don't know who they're sleeping with. The conversation to say 'this is not normal' has to start somewhere. And, as fun as it seems at the time that you're doing it, it's not serving us. It's fun until it's not fun.

Part Three

HOW WE'RE BEING PLAYED

17.

Big Alcohol

I have been writing about alcohol daily for more than eight years now, ever since I first quit drinking. That's one topic, every day for eight years. I can't begin to count the number of blogs, articles, Facebook updates, Instagram posts, tweets, presentations and speeches I have written and delivered on this one topic, not to mention the number of interviews and discussions I've had with journalists, presenters and podcasters. Hundreds, and in all of them I have trodden a very clear line, remaining concentrated on the personal process of getting sober and learning how to live alcohol-free. This is no accident—I have consciously maintained this personal and direct focus for a very good reason.

From the moment I decided to face up to my drinking problem and do something about it, I was very clear in thinking, *I can't change the world, but I can change me.* I decided on day one that the best place to direct all my energy and effort was not on the booze-soaked state of the world, but on myself. I was right to do that, because quitting booze took a lot of hard internal work, and the proof is in the pudding because here I am today living as a happy sober person! Over the years, as my recovery has become more solid and I haven't needed to put so much effort into fixing myself, I've redirected my energy into talking directly to others who are struggling with alcohol, but always still maintaining the same focus on the internal process of getting sober. Like I said before, this is no accident. I've chosen to focus on reaching people on a personal level, fearing that if I veer too sharply into the realm of feisty political speak I'll miss the opportunity to help others quit. I know from personal experience that, if you're in a dark and miserable place with booze, you're not likely to turn your life around by getting angry at the privileged position alcohol holds in society and the power the liquor industry wields. Fighting the big fight would take up so much energy there'd be little left to apply to yourself.

Maintaining this personal focus has meant that I've pretty much avoided any wider discussions around alcohol's status in society, the laws and regulations (or lack thereof) relating to this drug, or the lobbying and manipulation coming from the liquor industry (aka Big Alcohol). I haven't spent time highlighting how Big Alcohol is a multi-billion-dollar industry working determinedly in numerous sophisticated ways to ensure we remained liquored up.

I haven't talked about how lax liquor laws have enabled our booze-soaked culture, which in turn has escalated alcohol-related harm. I haven't complained about the almost unfettered access alcohol-industry lobbyists have to our lawmakers, how easily they are able to bend their ears and shower them with gifts.[1] Nor have I pointed out how uneven the playing field is, with public-health researchers, campaigners and officials not being afforded the same access to lawmakers or having the same lucrative coffers to draw from. I haven't complained about how easy it is for premises to get liquor licences, and how hard it is for them to lose them.

I haven't bemoaned how the industry spends huge amounts of money fighting legal battles with local governments and community groups that are desperately trying to push back and reduce alcohol-related harm without the same deep pockets.[2]

I haven't unpicked the ruthless sales and marketing tactics Big Alcohol uses to ensure high sales volumes, or complained endlessly (and it *would* be endless if I was to start) about all the ridiculously biased and misleading propaganda everywhere that glorifies alcohol while ignoring its many proven downsides. (Nor do I bemoan the loose advertising and sponsorship rules and regulations that allow these manipulative and untrue messages to keep being promoted.) I haven't pointed out how disingenuous and cynical it is for alcohol brands to align themselves with wellness events,[3] and mental health campaigns,[4] given the well-documented evidence of the emotional and physical harm their products cause to humans.

I haven't protested at how the industry denies and deliberately causes confusion about the irrefutable links between alcohol and cancer, and how they pay experts to lie and discredit scientific data showing otherwise. I haven't railed against any of the denials, omissions, distortions and distractions constantly spouted by industry spokespeople, including their most recent tactic, which is to encourage women to drink during pregnancy by publishing false and misleading information about the risks involved.[5] And I haven't pointed out the futility and harm caused by their endless focus on drinker education,[6] given that not only is there no evidence to show better education works to reduce consumption, but it completely ignores the fact that alcohol is an addictive drug and for many of us no amount of knowledge about how to moderately consume it is going to make a blind bit of difference.

Of all of these many troubling things about Big Alcohol, this last one in particular—the tactic of shining the spotlight endlessly on 'drinker education'—is the one that grates with me the most. I also believe it's the one aspect of the bigger picture that would actually be useful and empowering for people who are struggling with booze to understand.

The industry works very hard in this area because they know it makes them look good. They have websites devoted to drinker education,[7] they commission research into it,[8] they run workshops on it.[9] Their argument is that we'd all be better off if only we knew how to drink moderately, reasoning that if we had the correct information about things like standard drink sizes and safer drinking levels, we wouldn't run into trouble. It's heartbreakingly disingenuous.

Those who work in the field of public health and alcohol reform are well versed in this industry tactic of focusing on drinker education. Andy Towers, an Associate Professor at Massey University's School of Health Sciences, told me, 'As soon as you see an alcohol brand come out with any sort of alcohol-related public-health information, you know off the bat that they're going to be blaming the victim. They're going to be saying, "People don't know how to drink."'

Towers, a passionate campaigner for stronger public policies around liquor, explained to me how this 'victim blaming' tactic is a common one used by lobbyists worldwide, and not just those working in the alcohol sector. 'Just like the gun lobby says, "It's not about the guns; it's about the people who use them," the alcohol lobby says, "It's not about the alcohol; it's about the drinker." And what we know is that's complete rubbish. A lot of the reason people drink the way they do is because of the culture of drinking in a country and the social norms that have been developed.'

It also flies in the face of the fact that alcohol is an addict-ive drug that many people simply cannot moderate. As lawyer and alcohol campaigner Grant Hewison says, 'The focus on the individual doesn't work when addressing social issues like alcohol or gambling. It fundamentally doesn't work because these things are clearly addictive, and people can't moderate their behaviour because of the way addiction works in the brain.'

Big Alcohol doesn't see it this way of course, nor do they call what they do 'victim blaming'. They talk instead about 'personal responsibility'. This is their big thing. Always with the bloody 'personal responsibility'. But, like I say, it's disingenuous and insincere. They're ignoring the proven facts about this addictive drug, trying to make themselves look good while attracting attention away from their own ruthless and predatory sales behaviour. They want to make it appear as though they care about the high levels of alcohol-related harm in our communities, but they don't. I'll say it again and again and again to ram this point home: Alcohol is an addictive drug that many people, no matter how well informed they are, simply cannot moderate. By focusing on drinker education and personal responsibility, Big Alcohol is ignoring the statistics on how many hundreds of thousands of people struggle to control this addictive drug. They're also ignoring the rock-solid proof that the best way to change habits is not through education but through public policy.[10] But worst of all, in my opinion, their rhetoric around personal responsibility also serves to isolate and stigmatise people who are unable to moderate and control their intake. This is why those of us who struggle with alcohol need to be able to easily unpick this personal responsibility/drinker education bullshit rhetoric.

The alcohol industry's 'if only you knew more you'd be okay' approach makes those of us who struggle with this drug feel bad and weak, like it's some sort of personal failing that we can't control our intake. Because what they're basically saying is, 'Anyone can moderate if they have the right information.' And that simply isn't true. It certainly wasn't true for me. No amount of knowledge was going to magically make me want to stop drinking after one glass of wine. Understanding a standard drink size wasn't going to stop me pouring huge buckets of wine. Hearing recommended weekly limits wasn't going to stop me drinking every night. It might work for a few people—like Mandy, who shared her story earlier on page 60—but not all. My brain, like the brains of many others, is simply wired differently. We're wired to want more, more, more. That's addiction, folks.

But Big Alcohol's 'educational' approach doesn't allow for or even acknowledge my experience, or the experience of anyone who is remotely like me (very convenient if your business is in keeping people drinking). Rather, their approach works to keep us feeling stigmatised and isolated, like we're wrong for not being able to achieve something that we can't: moderation.

Take Olivia, for example. In her story, shared earlier on page 38, she was very honest about being worried that her drinking habit was dysfunctional and out of control. Yet despite numerous red flags (worsening hangovers, increased cravings, persistent guilt and mental-health struggles) she was still clinging to the belief that things could be different for her. 'I'd like to become a sensible drinker,' she said, and, 'I'm hoping that I . . . maybe leave alcohol for special occasions.' Her hope —that her relationship with alcohol could somehow magically be different from how it actually is—is fuelled by industry-pushed rhetoric that moderation is achievable for everyone through better education. They've been pushing this line so hard and for so long it has embedded itself into common parlance.

'It's a really difficult discourse to break,' Dr Nicki Jackson tells me. She's the executive director of Alcohol Healthwatch, an organisation dedicated to reducing and preventing alcohol-related harm in New Zealand. 'When we do our polling and we ask people why we should be taking action on alcohol, they all say, "Well it's just your personal responsibility." The person down the street doesn't see the problem with it. They think the individual should just be able to make those right choices.'

If only our collective discourse acknowledged that it's not simply a question of everyone making the 'right choices'. If only our collective discourse didn't buy what the liquor industry wants us to believe, but the truth. That is, that a large proportion of the population is—despite their best efforts—not able to moderate their intake.

If we did, as a society, outwardly acknowledge the fact that alcohol is an addictive drug and can't be moderated by everyone (and stopped allowing the industry to push the opposite line), then adopting the position that you're struggling would be much easier for people like Olivia and myself. But as it stands, with people buying the rhetoric that everyone should be able to moderate and control their intake (and better education is the key to getting them there), this personal responsibility line acts as a huge barrier to change. It also feeds into the stigma around addiction. 'It's hidden. It's taboo,' says Belinda, who also shared her story earlier, on page 84, 'and you're not allowed to admit it.'

So if you are struggling, and you hear an industry spokesperson pointing the finger at you, claiming you simply don't have enough knowledge to keep yourself under control, be aware that they're being arseholes. They're ignoring the cold, hard facts about alcohol, while working like demons to make themselves look good, maintain their profits and keep you drowning in a sea of booze, feeling weak and alone. They might wrap their actions and rhetoric in a shroud of care and responsibility, but make no bones about it—underneath, it's disingenuous, deeply damaging, misleading and insincere.

18.

Glenn

'They push their products. They push, they push, they push.'

My mum and dad drank, Dad particularly heavily. His drinking wasn't good—he'd get drunk and biff my mother around a bit. I can remember that as a very small child. I didn't drink until I was in my mid twenties because I had children very young—I got pregnant at sixteen. I had to marry the father but he wasn't a good man. He used to hit me like my dad hit Mum, so I walked out. I moved around a lot with the kids, and eventually moved up north and lived in a motor camp. The conditions were awful there.

I did have one very good friend in the motor camp, and he used to invite me over to drink. I can remember us counting out our money on the table for a half gallon of wine. I can taste it now—how revolting. I moved when I was around 30 to the house I'm still in now, and the people who lived around me used to get together and have a beer on a Saturday night. So I got into it more then—it turned into a bit of a party city. We used to be naughty and drink spirits and other stuff if we had enough money. It got a bit ridiculous because I got into a bit of debt.

I never drank every day, but did on payday and the weekends. I'd always have something on the stove to feed my children, but sometimes I couldn't remember putting them to bed, so it got a little bit messy. That went on for five years, then I got a bit concerned and thought, *This is ridiculous*, so I pulled myself together. It was going in a direction that was quite bad so I stopped altogether, cold turkey. I found a job then, as a teacher aide. I haven't touched alcohol now for twenty-odd years, largely because of the memory of my father and my mother. It still resonates in the back of my mind.

I'm 71 now. When I look around I see alcohol everywhere; it's not a good thing. They push their products. They push, they push, they push. It's in the papers, it's on TV, it's everywhere. Even in *Coronation Street* they're always drinking. At the supermarket they put the alcohol right opposite the fruit and veg. We teach the kids in school that five-plus a day is really good, but in the supermarket the veggies are all opposite the alcohol, just like it's lemonade. It breaks my heart when I see it. My community is scored as a ten on the New Zealand deprivation index, which means we're in the bottom ten per cent in terms of deprivation, but it's a fabulous community. I love living here. Everyone's very caring and loving, and it's very multicultural. The drums beat, the hula girls hula. We have lots of culture days, they're fabulous and the food is great. But there are liquor outlets everywhere. Within one kilometre of my house alone there are eight alcohol shops. We don't want them in our community—they're preying on the weak and the poor.

When I left work I really needed something else to do other than be in the house and quilt. So I got involved in a group that stopped a motorway being built. We banded together and fought Auckland Council and stopped it. One night at one of our meetings this lawyer guy, Grant Hewison, appeared to speak to us about alcohol. He said, 'I'll show you how to make oppositions to liquor licences and objections and all of that.' I thought he was an upstart lawyer—oh, I was angry. He used all these technical terms. I didn't know what he was talking about! I was only a girl from Mangere with limited education. But he came the following week, and the following week—he came three times to talk to us. He's so good; he taught us and got us organised. We learned how to put in objections, we learned how to go to a District Licensing Committee hearing. Our group is called Communities Against Alcohol Harm.

If an alcohol shop is going to start up, they have to apply for an off-licence to sell that alcohol. Before they can do that, they have to advertise in the paper that this is what they're going to do, and our group sees that and we oppose it. We say to them, 'No, we don't want you opening there because there's lots of schools around. We don't want you having any advertising on your windows or on your roof.' We put lots of conditions on and then we have a hearing with the District Licensing Committee. There's usually three people that sit on that—I think they're all either retired police officers or JPs or judges or something. The person who's applying for a licence, they have an expensive lawyer there, paid for by the alcohol industry.

When we first started, by golly, it was all uphill. We had no idea what we were doing. We'd sit there and maybe wee our pants a little because we were so scared. And they didn't listen to us; they thought that we were just a bunch of annoying people, in it for our own gratification. But, man, we hung in there. We hung in there and another year went past, and we hung in there. And all of a sudden we saw a change in their attitude and the way that they saw and spoke to us. It was nice and open, more respectful. Now I can go in, sit down and talk away, and it makes no difference to me because I realised that they're only people.

I've been doing this work for four years now. I've signed objections from a hospital bed, I've been part of big street protests. I get a buzz out of it all. It matters because a lot of the shop owners who want to sell alcohol don't care about our community. They don't care that there's lots of schools around and kids under eighteen will be walking past the doorway every day. They don't care that we're a low-decile area with people drinking all day and night. They don't care about all the terrible drinking that goes on—but I do. I find it really sad.

Lots of people say to us that it's amazing what we're doing, but we don't feel like that. We feel like we're just doing something that we've got time to do. And other people are a wee bit shy to do it. I do feel like we're fighting a losing battle a lot of the time, but I will never give up. Because there's a light at the end of the tunnel. Quietly, we're having an impact.

19.

Targeting women

It was Christmas Day and I was close to tears, hiding in the bedroom at my sister-in-law's house. I'd just been doing a quick check of my social-media accounts, and what I'd seen had filled me with despair. The first thing was a private Facebook message: 'Please, Mrs D, can you help? Alcohol is killing me, but I can't stop.' As often happens when I receive these sorts of messages (which is all the time), my heart ached for this woman I'd never met. I so clearly understood her pain. I knew exactly the miserable place she was in, how stuck she felt. I've been there and it's horrendous. I longed to help her get free. I typed out a quick reply, encouraging her to join our community at livingsober.org.nz, then flicked over to Instagram in the hopes of seeing something uplifting in my feed there. Instead I got hit with twisted lies.

One of the first images that showed up was of a glamorous and well-groomed woman smiling broadly at the camera, holding a flute full of sparkling white wine. An advert for a well-known wine company, with the caption reading something like 'The world is yours for the taking'. For Pete's sake! On top of the heartache I was feeling for the desperate woman who had just reached out to me, I was now hit by a wave of anger and frustration. The immense disconnect between the lies that are presented to us about women and alcohol and the reality as I was seeing it was so brutally apparent it made me want to weep. How could this wine company be allowed to push their bullshit out into the world? Why was this misleading propaganda allowed into my Instagram feed? I knew that, if I was seeing the ad, thousands of other women would be too—many feeling just like the one who had messaged me. Clearly *not* like the world is theirs for the taking. The manipulation was outrageous—they were selling an image that is so often miles away from the truth.

This manipulation of women by the liquor industry is not a new thing, of course. They've been doing it since forever. Even as far back as the start of last century, when men in New Zealand were boozing up large but women weren't actually drinking that much, alcohol barons were trying to mess with our heads. I recently found a propaganda poster from 1911 on which the National Council (a collection of hoteliers, alcohol producers and merchants) claimed that any woman voting in favour of prohibition was essentially weak and 'confessing their lack of influence over the hearts and minds of their men folk'.[1] We might not have been drinking much back then, but we did have the vote. The National Council taunting women to vote in their favour by accusing them of being weak if they didn't really was a dickhead move.

It was decades later, in the 1960s, when the liquor industry really started setting its sights on the female drinker. Until that point most alcohol marketing had been pitched firmly towards men, but adverts from the sixties show booze brands claiming their products would help relieve the boredom and sadness of women who were stuck at home all day while hubby was out at work. Images of glamorous and well-groomed women (of course) holding glasses full of wine were placed alongside slogans like 'To help you cope with life's little ups and downs' and 'Keep Calm and Banish Depression'.[2] 'It's alright for him,' goaded one particular advert, 'He goes off in the morning . . . but all you have is an empty house and the same dull rounds of household tasks. It's on days like this that "Sanatogen" Tonic Wine is so helpful.'

Women's Lib just got Big Alcohol even more jazzed about hooking us in. The more doors that opened in society for women, the more the liquor industry simply saw opportunities to increase their market share. 'I think the alcohol industry was possibly one of the first industries to jump onboard women's rights and see it as a way to advance their own cause and their own popularity,' Andy Towers from Massey University's School of Health Sciences told me. 'If women don't have to stay at home, if they can work, they can have careers, then they can play as hard as the boys. And if you're playing as hard as the boys, you really should relax like the boys, so here's a drink. It's a despicable way to hijack something that should be good, which is empowerment.'

Wine advertisements targeted at women around the late 1960s and the 1970s all projected an aura of sophistication, beauty, celebration and refined taste (those glamorous and well-groomed women again). But, just like the disconnect apparent today, the reality behind the myths didn't always match up. As Ruth admitted in her story earlier on page 113, in the 1980s, she and her friends saw getting trashed as somehow 'powerful'. But there were also 'hideous' times, 'vomiting and pissing yourself at the same time'. Not the sort of images you'd ever see in an advert promoting drinking.

Images of messy, drunk women weren't used by the spirits industry, either, when they launched alcopops in the early 1990s. These sweet, pre-mixed drinks were seen as a good way for spirits companies to get a slice of the female drinking market, particularly aimed at catching women when they were young. The marketing around these pre-mixed lolly drinks was overtly feminine, and once again pushed the vibe of fun, friendship and partying. It worked. By 2004 girls and women aged between 13 and 28 were the biggest consumers of these drinks.

Award-winning Canadian journalist Ann Dowsett Johnston documents the rise of alcopops in her part-memoir *Drink: The intimate relationship between women and alcohol*, claiming that the industry did what it set out to do, which was 'reach out to females, and establish a bridge to the parent brands like Smirnoff vodka and Bacardi rum'.[3] She also notes, 'And of course, none of the marketing shows the consequences of drinking.' The drunk teenager passed out on the street, the smashed twenty-something falling over in bars, the boozed housewife trying to vomit quietly into her toilet so the kids don't wake up (that was me *sad-face emoji*) . . . You don't see images like these splashed around, do you? Oh no, it's only ever the glamorous, well-groomed women happily drinking that make it onto the glossy ad.

Studies show there's been a clear feminisation of alcohol products since the 1990s.[4] And the tried-and-true technique used to entice women into drinking is of course claiming that drinking alcohol leads to a fabulous lifestyle: drinking apparently makes women happy, more attractive, less stressed and more sociable. Brands entice us to 'have it all' and 'take over the world'. Writing for The Temper, journalist Irina Gonzalez says the sexy, persuasive alcohol ads targeted towards women feed us the same story over and over again, which is: 'Drink and you will be happy.' She writes, 'Alcohol marketing tells us that this is what life is all about. It isn't.'[5]

Professor Carol Emslie heads up the Substance Use and Misuse research group at Glasgow Caledonian University and has spent years researching gender and alcohol use. 'There's been a move from campaigns in the past which would sexualise and objectify women to sell alcohol to men,' she tells me over the phone from Scotland, 'to campaigns now trying to link their brands with fun, sophistication, female friendship and, perhaps most worryingly, with empowerment.' To highlight the cynical linking of booze with female empowerment, Professor Emslie points out how the liquor industry has recently moved to align itself with the modern-day movements #metoo and #timesup. One beverage company released a sparkling wine in a can called #TimesUp on International Women's Day, the same day that Johnnie Walker released their limited-edition Jane Walker scotch, 'celebrating the many achievements of women'.

Of course there are many other drinks produced specifically with the female drinker in mind. Skinnygirl Cocktails, The Sisters, Babe, Girls' Night Out, Mommy's Time Out and

Mad Housewife wines are just a few examples. The packaging is often pink, the imagery fun and any woman pictured always looks (you guessed it) glamorous, happy and well groomed. There are also some hideous feminine products on sale designed to help women secretly drink. Tampon cases that hide mini bottles, hollow bracelets that are actually flasks, bras that conceal bladders of wine—they're all available online.

One new tactic being used by the liquor industry to target women is to align themselves with the clean-eating and wellness craze.[6] Look for anything with 'natural', 'low-carb' or 'organic' on the label. There are even wines being marketed as keto and paleo-friendly. Manufacturers know that it's women who are most likely to be swayed by the use of such language. One study into gender preferences in wine marketing found that, of all the many information cues people look for when purchasing a bottle of wine (such as colour, brand name or style of wine), the word 'organic' was the only one that women responded to in more significant numbers than men.[7]

Another thing the liquor industry loves to do is align itself with female-centric events, such as lifestyle expos, wellness retreats and women's triathlons (yes, really). I cringed recently when I saw that a wine company was one of the main sponsors of a well-being event being hosted by a women's magazine. 'I'm a woman who does extraordinary things, every day' said the slogan on their event merchandise, while the sponsor's wine bottles carried images of women jumping for joy. Special days in the calendar to celebrate women are also always pounced upon as good opportunities to boost alcohol sales. One of the 2019 official partners of International Women's Day was the multinational beer and spirits company Diageo. To mark their involvement they launched a series of videos with female employees talking about things like inclusion and balance.[8] I watched them all to see if they mentioned the misery and destruction their products cause for women worldwide. Surprise, surprise, they didn't.[9]

While many liquor companies launch special drinks to mark International Women's Day,[10] Mother's Day is also seized upon. I saw an awful ad in my Instagram feed on Mother's Day this year. A brewery was appealing to kids to buy their mother beer as a thanks for all her hard work: 'Say cheers to one of the greats this Mother's Day with a personalised box of Speight's,' they invited. I can think of many ways I'd like my sons to thank me for all the work I do for them. Scented candles, bath bombs, breakfast in bed, even just a big hug and a 'thanks, Mum!' would suffice. But a box of personalised beer? I'll pass. I'm particularly annoyed to think my fifteen-year-old might have seen this ad in his own Instagram feed, and be manipulated by its glossy appearance.

It's not just obvious sales and marketing tactics that are being used by the industry to manipulate women. Where they've become really clever is through analysing and understanding our shopping behaviours. According to industry insider Natalie, a feisty and impassioned former liquor sales executive who shares her personal story next, on page 138, it's gone far beyond blatant marketing ploys. 'Stuff like the flasks shaped like tampon cases, that's very gimmicky,' she tells me. 'That's not actually the big liquor companies doing that. They are very careful to be seen to be treading a line, but then they pay hundreds of thousands of dollars to re-create liquor-store setups, putting in test shoppers and using laser trackers to see where their eyes are scanning and how long it takes them to make a purchase—' I stop her mid-sentence. 'Laser trackers? Really?' Suddenly I feel even more manipulated than before. But Natalie leaves no doubt as to how deeply the industry has analysed the female consumer: 'They know that women generally make a purchase in under three minutes, that they generally will have between one and three children with them at the time. They know what price point they're looking for, they know where on the shelf to have it, they know what wording to use. They are much more advanced than making products that will fit casks of wine in them. They play in a whole other league.'

As horrendous as being profiled right down to our eye movements sounds, it's all above board. As Natalie points out, liquor companies are merely utilising technology to understand how to position their brands so that customers recognise and purchase them in minimal time. Many different companies and industries are doing that. The deeper problem when it comes to alcohol is that, on top of clever sales techniques, its manufacturers are also allowed to make all the wild marketing claims they like about the supposedly positive benefits of their products, while at the same time ignoring—or misleading about—the downsides. The only way to stop that and end the manipulation of women through misleading propaganda is to regulate against it. Make it illegal for liquor companies to make endless positive claims about their products and force them to label their products as inherently dangerous. Sadly, worryingly, frustratingly, this is not something my government, or the governments in any other booze-soaked countries, appear to be looking at doing any time soon.

20.

Natalie

*'I have never worked in a job that
was so isolatingly competitive.'*

I never saw a life without alcohol. I worked in pubs from the age of sixteen, and at 24 I was hired by one of the largest global liquor companies as a sales rep. I was so naïve. They would send me into small towns with big drinking problems. Some of these places were so rough, there would be drunk people passed out on the street at ten o'clock in the morning. They'd drop me in there once every two months to load up and make my targets, and the way that they spoke about the people we were selling alcohol to was horrific. They were just a cash cow. That was my induction into working in the liquor industry. It was pretty eye-opening.

In the liquor sales business, you're all selling identical products, and the only differentiating factor is the brand itself, so it's an incredibly competitive environment. The push from your employer is to win over publicans by drinking and partying with them, all on the corporate card and often outside of work hours. They look for a certain type of salesperson—I can see that in hindsight. Someone in their early to mid twenties, channelling a kind of party vibe, but still looking quite healthy. That was definitely me at the time. I was drinking really heavily, but I was still young enough that I could do that and turn up to work the next day.

After a couple of years I was headhunted by a big global liquor company. That was even more of a work hard, play hard culture. A week after I started we flew away on a vineyard tour. I was with a group of guys, because the liquor industry is very blokey, and it was an anything-goes culture—shots of tequila at ten-thirty in the morning type of thing. We got totally hammered on our first night there, and they all talked the barmaids into coming back to their hotel rooms. My read from that was if I wanted to be part of the group I needed to participate in that behaviour. My drinking escalated really quickly. Every Friday at midday we'd start drinking, under the guise of it being educational, and then unbelievably we'd all drive home. That still blows my mind.

I worked there for a couple of years, then relocated back to my home town. I was in my late twenties, working two jobs in the liquor industry—one during the day, one at night. Both were alcohol-soaked environments that escalated my drinking even more. I started to really isolate and drink quite heavily at home by myself, after work and on days off, every time into a blackout. I knew it was a problem, but I had so completely lost perspective of what was normal. I kidded myself that everyone else was doing it as well.

I started working for yet another powerhouse global liquor company. I have never worked in a job that was so isolatingly competitive. The bonuses were massive, more than people's salaries, and I'd go to work knowing there were 100 people they could replace me with tomorrow. I'd come home from work every day and completely write myself off. I had shocking anxiety, really bad—panic attacks while driving sort of thing—probably to do with my drinking as well. I didn't go to a doctor because I didn't want them to ask me about alcohol. People were trying to help me and I would just burn them. You create your own narrative in those situations, just to get through. As soon as I thought, *I've got to make some changes*, I would get so overwhelmed with the shame of where I was that I would write myself off again. I felt like I'd got what everyone told me was success, but it was just so lonely and shit. It makes me angry that I fell for it.

Things eventually got so bad I quit my job, left everything behind except my dog, and moved to the other side of the country. I got a job outside of the liquor industry, but was still drinking every day and really struggling. I was so thin because I wouldn't have dinner; I'd just have two bottles of wine and half a pack of cigarettes. It was awful. I was 'that girl' who'd had a fabulous career but blown it up. It was like a really shit Hollywood movie. And I'm well read—I should have at least been like a Tolstoy tragedy, not like a freaking Netflix drama.

I recognised, at least in my subconscious, that I had a serious problem. I think I was in the precontemplation stage of getting sober. I started trying crazy things to control my intake, like pouring out half a bottle of wine before I started drinking so I'd only be able to have two glasses. But then I'd get in the car and drive to the bottle store to buy another bottle. I changed my life in other ways, in the great hope that I'd discover that alcohol wasn't the problem. So I was like, 'I'm turning celibate because maybe it's men. I do love the bad boy—maybe this is why I'm setting my life on fire.' No, that didn't make everything better. 'Maybe I should start running?' That didn't make everything better. 'Maybe I should learn Italian?' That didn't make everything better. 'Maybe I should eat more broccoli?' That didn't make everything better.

Then, in December 2015 I just got to a point where I had had enough. So I stopped drinking. I detoxed on my bathroom floor, and it was freaking horrendous. That was three and a half years ago now and I haven't had a drink since.

I love it. I love it so much. It's done wonders for my life. I've learned that I am a massive introvert. I am a cup-of-tea-drinking, stay-at-home, play-with-my-dogs, read-a-book type of girl. I think at heart that was always me. I never wanted a crazy career, but you buy into that lifestyle. I'm not saying that I shouldn't have opened my eyes more, but I was eighteen when *Sex and the City* was big. I was of that generation where you could have a career and lots of cocktails, and it was completely condoned and encouraged by the liquor industry I worked in. When I was 24 my bonuses were like twenty thousand dollars. It was a crazy, grand lifestyle, but in hindsight some of the practices that I engaged in were pretty morally ambiguous, to say the least.

I've been really public about stopping drinking and I've had so many people contact me, some of whom are former colleagues still in the liquor industry. They get in contact either to say 'well done', or frighteningly more often, 'I'm really struggling, can you help?' I've found that very challenging, because I don't think I've ever made even one good enough life decision for anyone to follow my example. But I'll answer people's questions. I say, 'I've been there, this is what I did to move on, and it doesn't make me a bad person.'

I can remember being in my backyard alone with a glass of wine, trying to make myself say, 'I am an alcoholic.' I was terrified. I couldn't say it in the privacy of my own backyard. And now I can. Now I'm like, 'Yeah I'm an alcoholic, and I'm also hot and I'm funny and I'm a dog mom and I'm a sister and a daughter.' It's just one label.

21.

Warrior Mums
of the world, unite

Isn't social media lovely? So safe and kind, full of positivity and connectedness, where people share only truthful and uplifting content based on good intentions and solid information. Yeah, right. The truth about social media, as we all know, is that it's a deeply complex and conflicted arena. It can bring joy and connectedness, but, boy, can it also bring pain and negativity. At best we get to enjoy highlights from our loved ones' lives, and access useful and interesting content from individuals and organisations we choose to follow. At worst, we get all manner of stuff that can make us feel isolated, upset, jealous, worried and angry. Nowhere is that more apparent than when it comes to alcohol-related content.

There is a veritable crap-tonne of booze-related material floating around social media. Most of it is targeted at women, especially mums. We seem to be ripe for the picking when it comes to online alcohol promotion. Quirky memes with vintage cartoon images chirp 'Motherhood: Powered by love, fuelled by coffee, sustained by wine' and 'Wine is to women what duct tape is to men: it fixes everything'. Photoshopped images show mums guzzling from ginormous wine glasses under the words 'I wish my tolerance for my children would increase as much as my tolerance for wine' and 'Tick-tock it's wine o'clock'. Babies are snapped wearing onesies with slogans saying 'I'm the reason mum drinks'. Cutsie nicknames for alcohol like 'mummy's juice' or 'mummy's little helper' get liberally bandied about. This is the Wine Mum culture online and it's rampant. Images are liked, shared and commented on at such a rate they've spread around platforms like Facebook, Instagram, Twitter, Pinterest and Snapchat like the plague.

'There was a time when "mummy needs wine" jokes were genuinely a little subversive,' writes *Metro* magazine in an advice column. 'Joking about needing a drink because your kids are driving you insane was once a kind of shorthand for communicating something difficult in a lighthearted manner, because life is hard and being a parent is extra hard and sometimes it's good to acknowledge that in a way which doesn't feel relentlessly negative.'[1] But, the magazine notes, the tone has now shifted: 'In its relentless quest to wring each last drop of utility from every pop culture phenomenon, the internet rewards the retelling of the same joke until it's flattened and wrung dry.'

What once offered a cheeky laugh has now been bastardised and cynically commercialised to the point where it's simply no longer funny. The once subversive little in-joke is now a deafening roar, and we can't hear ourselves think (let alone parent) without being hit with the message that we need alcohol to help us carry out our motherly duties. We'd all still be laughing if it wasn't so bloody damaging.

Being a mum is wonderful, but it's also hard work on so many levels. Births can be traumatising, sleeplessness is crippling, hormone surges are overwhelming, information overload is intense, insecurity hobbles us, opinions come from everywhere, cabin fever is real and loneliness sometimes achingly painful. Having a drink at the end of a long and tiring day can offer us a way out, and I've been very open about the fact that my drinking escalated hugely when I started being at home more after having kids. Opening a bottle of wine at 5 p.m. made me feel like I was still participating in the 'adult world'; taking the first sip flooded my body with dopamine and took the edge off my *insert any tricky emotion you can think of here*. I was drinking alone, but there's no doubt I felt supported and encouraged in my solo habit by all the Wine Mum content pouring from my computer. It helped me justify my regular, heavy drinking. It normalised it, and it made me feel connected with other mums who were dealing with the same shit (literally, at times) as I was, in the same liquid way.

'"Wine mom" culture was a blast for problem drinkers like me,' Halley Bondy writes on The Temper. 'I was a brand-new mom when the Internet started chanting, "Rosé all day!" I was there on the front lines slurring, "Yes, way!" The memes, hashtags, mimosa brunches, and Insta pics of moms drinking cocktails to deal with their kids—they were enabling me and I loved it.'[2] Did I, Halley, or any of the thousands of other mums drinking our way through the days ever pause to fully contemplate who was generating a large proportion of this social-media content (the liquor industry), the cynical reason they were pushing it out across cyberspace (to promote their products and increase their profits), and what their messages were actually saying to us (that we weren't fit to handle motherhood without regular doses of liquid drugs, and that our kids were so intrinsically awful we needed to blur our brains to cope with them)?

Anna, who shares her story with us on page 175, reads very clearly the underlying message we're sending every time we click, like, comment and share. 'It's really sad. You're putting on Facebook about how you can't cope with everything so you're taking drugs. We're saying, "Look at us, we fall apart at the end of the day, we can't cope."'

Joanna, whose story you'll hear next, on page 149, also reads the messages loud and clear and it grates: 'I hate with a passion that whole thing of "wine o'clock". I just hate it. I see so many women I know on social media posting about their drinks, and I just think, *Do you not get what you are promoting here?* Maybe it's okay for them. But then most of the ones who put those photos up online, I know that they're not okay.'

And therein lies the problem with the Wine Mum culture. It masks the truth. It makes light of something that is often very heavy. It sells the idea that all is fun and laughter when it comes to mums and alcohol, when often it's anything but. It creates the illusion that everyone is having an uproariously great time on the wines, when in truth we're not. And, most damaging of all, it isolates mums who are struggling.

If you're feeling even slightly conflicted or worried about your drinking, or you're someone who is newly sober and emotionally fragile, there's nothing more confronting and isolating than seeing a bunch of photos and posts singing the praises of booze.

It can really mess with your head. If you're even slightly on the outside of the boozy vibe, Wine Mum content only serves to make you feel like a lonely, miserable loser. The posts that might have once made you feel amused and included can very quickly turn sour and begin to impact on you in a negative way.

When I first quit drinking and was hellishly vulnerable and raw, being on social media was hugely problematic. I'd spot a glossy photo depicting happy mums raising their glasses under the caption 'And on Wednesdays we drink wine' and I'd feel the sharp barbs of aloneness. A cartoon meme chirping 'The most expensive part of having kids is all the wine you have to drink!!' would stab like a knife. (Somehow the meme format with professional-looking illustrations and fonts made me feel particularly on the outside of the joke.)

Now that I'm solidly sober, it's much easier to read into and dismiss social media's alcohol-related content for what it is—a curated, distorted, narrow, manipulative and sometimes outright dishonest version of reality (more on that in chapter 23). But if you're not in that solid place, if you're feeling fragile, lonely or low (which, let's face it, many mums are at times for a multitude of reasons), it's super easy to be negatively impacted emotionally. It's super easy to forget that much of what we see on social media isn't real. It's super easy to take in just the surface 'funny ha ha' messages and not properly register the more destructive, isolating and hurtful messages underneath. And it's super easy to forget that we're goddam warriors who already have everything it takes to be kick-arse mums inside of us.

Yes, the days are long and hard and we often feel isolated, irrelevant, exhausted, bored and a million other tricky emotions—but, ladies, we've got this. We can do motherhood without copious amounts of wine. We don't need to guzzle a liquid drug that blurs our brains, numbs our emotions and disconnects us from our children, our partners and ourselves. We don't need to model to our kids that the only way to cope with them (and with life) is by drinking every night. We don't need to keep sharing content that pokes fun at our drunkenness while sending underlying messages that we're incapable of parenting in the raw. We don't need to make a show of everything being light, and we can instead embrace gloriously messy imperfection. We don't need to 'smooth the edges' and can instead relish our bumpy emotional landscapes. And we certainly don't need to keep sharing content that promotes the products sold by an industry that cares only about its profits, not empowering women to be their best selves. We are not Wine Mums; we're Warrior Mums—strong, courageous, dedicated, hardworking, vulnerable, resilient and capable. Go stick that on a meme.

22.

Joanna

*'I hate with a passion that whole thing
of "wine o'clock". I just hate it.'*

I wasn't allowed alcohol growing up. It was consumed quite freely by Mum and Dad, but I don't remember either of them ever being drunk, and we were certainly never given tastes of it. It was a reasonably strict upbringing and alcohol was a no-no for us.

I started drinking quite early, and Mum and Dad would have had a fit if they'd known what I was doing, so I hid it. I'd stay out at friends' houses instead of being at home so that my parents didn't have to see it. I was one Joanna at home, sitting at the dinner table, and another Joanna who went out and got plastered.

When I drank, I drank. You'd never see me have just two drinks. I absolutely loved drinking; I loved the freedom it gave me to essentially be someone else and be bold. I wasn't that person, and I'm still not that person. I'm probably quite introverted, but alcohol made me open up and be the social butterfly that I'm really not at heart. I was looking for approval and attention and love, and the bottom of a bottle wasn't the best place to look for that, but that's how I went about it.

There was a period in my twenties when I was binge drinking, but it wasn't an everyday occurrence and I still functioned quite well. I wouldn't say I was a healthy drinker then, but it was about weekend socialising, not having to have one, two or three bottles of wine at the end of each day. That came later on.

I went into a career in hospitality and got married and had two daughters. Still a big drinker but managing it. I think there was a part of me that knew that it was the only way I could connect with people, because the friends I had, all we did was drink. That's all we really had in common.

I lived with guilt for so many years. Like, *Did I bathe my kids last night? I can't really remember. Did I feed them? Did I put their chicken nuggets in?* (Because that's all they ever got when I was drinking.) But despite the guilt I still thought it was just fun.

By my mid thirties I was drinking daily, and it was heavy. Like, not just a couple of drinks daily; it was a lot daily. I was starting to have conflict with myself. I knew I wasn't happy. I wasn't happy with who I was, I wasn't happy in my marriage (which was largely because of who I was). I knew I was just trying to dull all of the questions that were coming up in me about facing up to life. My business was failing, it was swallowing money that I didn't have, and I started to hate people. When they walked in the restaurant door I really just wanted to tell them to fuck off. Not really conducive to running a good restaurant. Life was shit, and so I just drank and drank and drank.

I crashed my car once, drink driving. It was after a boozy lunch at my workplace and an afternoon of drinking. My colleagues tried to get my keys off me, but I managed to find them and get in my car, which was a Mini, and drive home. I must have blacked out, drove through a 'keep left' sign, over a traffic island and ripped the bottom of the Mini out. Fortunately my sister lived just up the road, so I managed to crawl the car into her driveway. I didn't go to work the next day because of the feeling of shame.

I was never once questioned over how much I drank. Nobody ever pulled me aside and said, 'Do you think you need to look at this?', because it's so accepted. And you can't tell me people didn't know how much I was drinking. I got drunk at family occasions. I got drunk everywhere, and it's okay, it's just okay. No one sees it as a drug, no one sees it as a poison. It's just what we do. 'Come on, we're Kiwis.'

I will say this. I am very lucky to have not been raped and I'm very lucky that I'm alive. Walking home drunk at night, sleeping in the bushes, all those things that I did. One night I stayed out after work, drinking a lot. I left very early in the morning, and there were no taxis around so I started walking home—drunk, oblivious, totally stripped down. A police van picked me up and the cop said he'd stopped me because he'd been watching a guy watching me and he didn't like the look of him. I was totally unaware.

I separated from my husband and was trying to get

sober but wasn't truly committed. I wasn't ready to live life without it yet, but I knew it was creating havoc. I attended an awards evening one night and drank myself into oblivion. I was in what had become a normal state of functioning—that is, an almost blackout state—when I suddenly realised I was back home and had brought with me a man who I knew to be married with children. I was mortified and disgusted in myself, threw him out, locked the door and sobbed hysterically. The next day was my sister's fortieth and I was supposed to go to a concert with her that night. I had to tell her I couldn't make it. I couldn't go into work either. Not because I was too hungover—I had worked through many, many hangovers over the past ten years—but because I was truly ashamed of myself and had come to realise that I had hit rock bottom with my drinking. This was it. I was officially recognising myself as an alcoholic.

Once the confidence alcohol gave me was gone I had to learn how to deal with who I am without it. I care about things a lot more now than I did then, because it was just easier to not question stuff, not question anything, just exist and laugh and be the girl who dances on the bar and entertains people. But I destroyed a lot of my friendships because of my drinking, and others didn't like me once I stopped. I can't do bullshit and I can't do small talk. It's not real because it's got this little film of alcohol that makes everything convivial. It feels real but it's dangerous. I made connections that weren't real for so long, I only want real now.

I have made some really good friendships with people who have only known me as sober Jo, which is nice. I don't think they'd like the other Jo, so that's quite cool. But I'm still quite reclusive, and I do find it hard to make new female friends without drinking. With other parents it's their automatic assumption that you drink, so they're like, 'We'll do drinks,' or, 'Let's catch up and have a wine.' I feel like it's a real effort for them to meet me because it's just going to be for coffee, but then I'll see them with other women and it's all about drinking. They're sharing photos on Facebook with drinks in their hands and I'm never getting invited into that situation. Maybe they feel I wouldn't enjoy it, which isn't true! Because I'm from hospitality, I'm the first one to pour a wine for someone if I see you with an empty glass. Or maybe they feel challenged having me there because they feel judged. Hey, I'm not judging you; this is only about me. This is totally just my journey. I don't give a shit what you do. I turned up once for a fundraising meeting and when they brought out the wine I said, 'Oh, no thanks, I don't drink,' and their reaction was quite deflated. I think I ruined the moment for them a little bit, crushed the expectation because of course everyone assumes that we all drink.

I hate with a passion that whole thing of 'wine o'clock'. I just hate it. I see so many women I know on social media posting about their drinks, and I just think, *Do you not get what you are promoting here?* And then I think, *Am I being biased because I've been through it and I've got to the other side?* Maybe it's okay for them. But then most of the ones who put those photos up online, I know that they're not okay.

I'm still a work in progress, even after more than eleven years sober. I always will be. But what I've learned about myself is huge. I've realised that I actually had no clue whatsoever about what was going on in my head and in my heart. Alcohol stopped me having to acknowledge anything about myself that was wrong or missing. I didn't acknowledge anything until I stopped drinking. I just thought life was a bit problematic; there was no self-awareness whatsoever. None. I look back at the boozy me now and feel so sad for her, realising how lost she was and how alone she was. So alone. Surrounded by people but alone. No real friends. She was just a lonely person who didn't really like herself. It was my mask, my coping mechanism.

I don't think of it as having given up alcohol; I think of it as having gained my life back. I have never loved life and all the people in my life like I do now.

23.

#dontpinkmydrink

If only we had a 'truth filter' or a 'full-story filter' to reveal the reality behind social-media images. Because, for the vast majority of the content we see online, all is not as it seems. First off, all the boozy party pics or 'here's me relaxing with alcohol' photos shared by ordinary people (i.e. not professional influencers, organisations or businesses) are often a little disingenuous. They're not necessarily outright false or deceitful, but they are curated to a certain extent and therefore only offer a fraction of the full picture. We all do it. We snap a bunch of photos, choose the best one, crop out distracting or unattractive background items and then slap on a filter to elevate the mood. Full context is seldom given; we only ever provide a narrow view of what's going on.

The 'I deserve this!' Instagram caption under your friend's glistening glass of chardonnay doesn't mention the tension you know she's experiencing in her marriage. The 'Fun with the girls!' group shot shared on Facebook by an ex-colleague doesn't highlight the seven tricky human emotions currently being experienced by the group. Who's sharing selfies of themselves in bed at 3 a.m. when they're full of guilt and remorse? I never did. Who's writing posts at 10 a.m. when their anxiety is peaking? Not many. That's not the stuff we tend to put online. We don't share when we're low; we wait until we're feeling fine again (perhaps when we've just had that lovely dopamine hit from the first glass of wine), and before you can say 'Clarendon' we're back on social media filtered to the hilt, once again showing our cheery face to the world, adding to the impression that all is rosy (or should that be rosé?) in the world.

Sober people aren't immune to this inadvertent deception. Just last week I celebrated my eight-year soberversary and proudly celebrated the milestone in posts on Facebook, Instagram and Twitter. I talked about how happy and proud I felt while sharing flattering photos of myself smiling widely. But my truth was far more complex. Yes, I was happy and proud about being eight years sober, but I was also stressed from writing this book, worried about some pending medical results, angsting over technical issues at livingsober.org.nz and exhausted from not sleeping well. Did any of my soberversary posts reflect those things? No. What I presented was a true *aspect* of my current human experience—I was proud and happy about reaching eight years sober—but it was just a fraction of the full range of emotions I was experiencing at the time. I was inadvertently deceiving by omission, presenting only a sliver of reality, which is all any of us can ever offer when we're sharing online. It pays to remember this, but that's easier said than done if you're sitting on your sofa with your phone in hand feeling low and vulnerable.

Even harder to unpick is all that alcohol-related content coming from the big players inside the liquor industry. These guys are bloody good at styling and manufacturing content for maximum effect, and they have expert teams working with mega-budgets. Not only do they know how to curate the slyest and most persuasive content, pushing it out without us knowing where it comes from, but also they know exactly how to use algorithms to target us.

Brydie Meinung is a social marketing expert—there's nothing about algorithms and social-media technologies she doesn't know—and she admits to me it's scary the extent to which we can be picked off and targeted. 'I don't think people really understand how deep it is. I think they understand that there is targeting going out, but I don't think they realise to what extent.'

Meinung spends her days helping people get their messages out on social media to exactly the audience they want. 'Not only can we target people based on whether they use Visa or Mastercard, what kind of car they drive, whether they have newborns or toddlers or teenagers or whether they're single, married or divorced, but also we can get even more specific by taking real data. Say a business has a database full of real people's email addresses; we can load in a whole lot of those that we know belong to women aged between 25 and 55, and the social-media platforms can then extrapolate that population out, find their profiles on Facebook or Instagram and then find other profiles that have very, very similar behaviours—liking the same pages, liking the same content—and target them.'

Yes, that's right. If you're sitting on your sofa, newly divorced, having just commented on an article about menopause in a private Facebook group, it's no accident that you start seeing ads in your feed for a bubbly wine promising to 'add a touch of sparkle to your life'. Meinung says it's impossible to hide. 'It is really hard to get away from it. We're also now targeting people on social media based on their activity on the normal web. So if they're on a certain website, looking at a certain type of shoe, they can literally go to their social media a couple of seconds later and see an ad with the exact pair of shoes, even though they've never looked at those products or that company on social media.' Yes! I just had that exact thing happen to me! I just googled 'collagen beauty powder' on my laptop (don't judge) and five minutes later opened Instagram on my phone, and lo and behold there was a bunch of adverts in my feed for various collagen products. That is super creepy.

What's even creepier is how big liquor brands are no longer relying solely on paid advertising and algorithms to get their message out. The new way they market on social media is by using professional influencers—people with massive amounts of followers getting paid to feature products and services in their posts. 'Brands have figured out that this is actually a better way of doing things,' Meinung tells me. 'They've said, "We don't need to put advertising through social-media platforms anymore. We can just get someone who looks pretty to endorse our product and make it look like your life can be like this if you have our drink." And these influencers or bloggers claim a very big market share of eyeballs on their content.'

Meinung points out that all of this online behaviour is above board. 'We're all just using the social-media platforms and the technologies within them that are available to everyone. It's not always harmful. But I do think that when the product being promoted is inherently damaging, like alcohol is, it does become problematic.'

Industry insider Natalie, who shared her story earlier on page 138, concurs. 'It's next level and it's so scary. It's not sparkly-eyed twenty-year-olds on a Midori billboard; it's an Instagrammer who you don't know being paid to advertise because they've got a glass of champagne in their hand. It's subliminal marketing and it's fucking with people's heads. They have "brand ambassadors" and they pay them to influence via social media. It's the predatory nature of that that probably terrifies me more than anything.'

If you take into account algorithms, the rise of brand ambassadors and influencers, and just the immense reach that platforms like Facebook, Instagram, Twitter, Pinterest, LinkedIn, YouTube and Snapchat have, you can see why these platforms have become 'important actors in the development of alcohol marketing techniques' (as one study says).[1] The liquor industry is creaming itself over the ease with which these platforms are helping them get their propaganda into people's personal spaces, combined with the fact there are very few regulations preventing them from doing and saying whatever they like. And who's on social media the most? Women.[2] And who's most likely to make a purchase based on content they see on social media? Women.[3]

So adept are liquor companies at targeting women on social media that an online campaign in the form of a hashtag has been launched by a group of alcohol and gender researchers at Glasgow Caledonian University. It's called #dontpinkmydrink. If you search it on Twitter you'll see it being used on a raft of images from all over the world, each one highlighting how alcohol brands are cynically marketing alcohol to women, piggybacking on empowerment movements and natural female camaraderie to sell their products.

I spoke with Professor Carol Emslie, who spearheads the initiative, and she told me, 'We want the campaign to raise awareness. All you might need is a little nudge to make you think it actually isn't great that we're all sharing content saturated with images of having a drink as a reward or being vital to female friendship. It's so normalised that until you take a step back it's almost quite hard to see it.'

The #dontpinkmydrink campaign is fairly new but Professor Emslie is hoping it will soon take off. 'We're really keen for it to be picked up more widely, rather than just among researchers and alcohol charities. We'd love for it to grow at the grassroots level, for women themselves to be talking about it and using it.' Particularly, she says, given Big Alcohol's huge marketing push towards women, which will only keep getting stronger. 'There's a real awareness in the alcohol industry that women are an important market, one that's not yet saturated. There's still more work to be done in targeting women as far as the alcohol industry is concerned.'

So the next time you're sitting on your sofa feeling low and lost, and you spot a Wine Mum meme or cynical marketing message linking alcohol to female empowerment, slap a #dontpinkmydrink hashtag on it before sharing it with your followers or friends. That's a genuinely empowering and satisfying move. A feisty little push-back to show we're not patsies being blindly manipulated; we can see through cynical marketing ploys and we're not having a bar of it. We know that any alcohol-related content attempting to unite women in rousing and empowering ways is actually faux camaraderie playing us for fools. We're not fools, so #dontpinkmydrink, thank you very much.

24.

Staci

'Until you stop doing it, you don't actually know how much it's impacting you.'

My mother had a serious problem with alcohol, so I grew up with a lot of drinking and parties around. It was just a normal part of our lives. But my mum was not a happy drunk, so the parties always ended up with drama and something bad happening. She left when I was twelve and moved up to Auckland, and I stayed behind with my dad. Her leaving had quite a significant effect on me, as I was at a pivotal point in my development, so that really impacted how I felt about myself. I felt like I was abandoned and unloved.

I came up on a holiday to visit her once with a friend. My mother was busy so she organised for this guy in his early twenties and his younger brother to take us out for the day. We thought this was amazing because we were pretty boy-crazy, and we pretended to be all sophisticated and mature. We visited a park and one of the guys offered me a beer. I didn't think my mother would have an issue with it, and didn't think about any consequences. I drank the beer straight away, just to be cool and to fit in. And my friend drank a little bit of hers, but she felt quite sick so she passed it on to me and I drank it back quickly. It was like a switch had been turned on in my head—I felt amazing. It was like, *This is what I've been looking for*. It made me feel happy and confident and like I was having fun, all the things that I wanted. All my problems were covered up, and I didn't feel scared or worried anymore. I just felt amazing, like I was free and alive.

Because I felt so bad normally, it was such a contrast to suddenly feel amazing. And, of course, because I only had one and a half beers, it wasn't enough to get any of the negative effects, just the positives, so that was forever linked in my brain. From then on I chased any opportunity to feel like that. But I never got it again really.

Dad didn't really drink, but he never challenged me on it that much. On a Sunday morning, if I'd come home drunk the night before, he'd get up in the morning and slam doors and make lots of noise and be annoying, and I think that was his way of acknowledging that he knew. He did sit me down once to say he was concerned about my drinking, mainly because of my mother—obviously he knew about that—but that was as far as it ever went. He never said 'you can't drink' or 'you shouldn't be drinking' or 'no, you can't go out'. He never had any rules, so basically I could just do whatever I wanted. No curfew, no restrictions or anything.

So without having boundaries I just went for it. Once I had that connection of how amazing alcohol made me feel, I wasn't going to not do it.

By fifteen I was out clubbing whenever I stayed with my mum, and at home she'd give me vodka. I didn't like her drinking. She'd be quite nasty when she was drunk and say really awful, horrible things to me about people in the family and stuff. But in the morning she'd just wake up pretending nothing had happened. There was a short period when I lived with her alone, and in the evening she would get drunk, vomit and pass out and I would have this terrible fear of not knowing what to do if she woke up. How was I going to look after her? But she'd just wake up and pretend everything was fine.

At parties I'd start out drinking and being happy, but because I had all these underlying emotional issues, I'd end up getting depressed and angry. I was really jealous and unable to control my emotions, so there'd be arguments and friends would have to go looking for me. Just drama, drama everywhere. This continued right through my teenage years.

At eighteen I moved up to Auckland on my own and started going to nightclubs and having random hook-ups. I really embraced being this strong, powerful, independent woman in the city. But in reality I just kept behaving in a way that made me feel more and more shameful and guilty and awful about myself. I hated myself so much, had even lower than the lowest self-esteem. I always felt alone and not connected with anybody, and was just looking for love and approval. When I went out and drank I felt confident, sexy and powerful. But it only lasted for a short time because by the next morning I felt really bad again. That feeling of shame is awful to live with.

I met my husband when I was twenty and managed to hide my drinking from him in those initial stages, because we were dating and not living together. When we did start living together we had parties, but all our friends were big drinkers too. It was that time in life when everyone did drink a lot, but I always took it a little bit too far.

Then my mother, who had gone to Africa, came home and was only back for two months before she passed away. I was 23 and that was the catalyst for sending me into a major spiral in my drinking. I just completely gave up any semblance of control and was in this really, really dark place. My husband and I got married a year after mum died, and we'd only been married for about six months when I hit rock bottom.

It was an awful week of drinking and drama, which ended with me on the bathroom floor, sobbing. I was in such a dark place and could not see any way out. In that moment I was completely suicidal—death was the only way I could see that I could get out. I prayed—cried out, really—and I believe God came and saw me, not physically, but I had a moment of inspiration and felt a little spark of hope rise in me. It was an encounter I suppose. And, for me, I felt like God was there with me in that room. And I suddenly thought, *There is a chance*. I felt hope rise in me that I could do it. I got off the floor, and haven't had a drink since.

It was a hard journey. The one thing I regret is not actually getting any counselling or treatment. I just stopped drinking and went to church, and yes a lot of healing happened in that process, but I didn't necessarily address the core issue, so that led on to other things. I took more prescription painkillers than I should have, and used food and other things to cope, rather than actually dealing with the issues. So it took me a while to learn how to sit with the pain. I think if I'd gone into treatment at the beginning, or had some professional help, maybe I would have learned that quicker. I've had loads of counselling since those early days. Talking to a professional was really helpful, because they were looking from the outside, so they could see things, patterns of behaviour, that I could not see.

I grew up with no boundaries. What I really needed was someone to tell me 'no'. I needed a safe place to fall. I say to people now, 'Don't be your kid's cool friend. Be a parent.' Alcohol and drugs are common and our kids are exposed to them at school, much younger than you would expect. Be aware and don't put your head in the sand. And be a good role model—teach your kids they can have fun without alcohol and show them how. You can't expect your kids to go to a party and have a good time not drinking if you, the parent, can't do that. Kids are more likely to copy your behaviour than your words.

When I was young and drinking, it was still kind of frowned upon for girls to get messy drunk, but now we see far more of it in our culture. For young girls it's almost seen as empowering or a rite of passage to get blotto drunk. And for many women on social media it seems to actually be something that they're proud of, that they need a wine to get through the day. I have a number of friends who will make comments about how much they need wine. It's a joke, but it seems to me like a weird thing to boast about.

I think that people have this impression that you can't have a good time without drinking. I see that a lot. It really scares me, the number of people who have a reliance on it and don't realise that they do. Sometimes, until you stop doing it, you don't actually know how much it's impacting you. When I was drinking I wasn't making decisions based on what I wanted. I was making them based on the feelings that I had—the shame and the guilt and feeling bad about myself—not from a place of power. That's all changed now.

Part Four

WHAT LIES BENEATH

25.

Liquid courage

There are a million reasons why women drink, but underlying all of them is this one: alcohol works. It would be stupid to deny this. Alcohol does what we want it to in the moment. When that liquid enters our bodies, gets carried around by our blood, hits our brains and triggers all those lovely chemicals, it feels good. We're instantly warmed, relaxed, uplifted, loosened and confident. Who wouldn't want that? That's the reason why so many of us drink. That's the reason why so many of us keep drinking even when there are negative impacts. Because, in that moment when we take that first sip, the drug works. It works.

Of course, the feelings aren't genuine. They're chemically induced, and once the drug departs our system we get dumped back down to our normal state (or lower than normal if we've been drinking a lot and our brain receptors have downregulated) and any uncomfortable emotions and insecurities are still there. But hey, take another drink and whammo! You're back in that lovely warm, relaxed and confident state.

Of all the feelings I've heard people say alcohol gives (or gave) them, this last one—confidence—is undoubtedly one of the most common. Time and again when people explain why they drink (or drank) alcohol they talk about it making them feel confident. On page 188 Charmaine admits that when she started drinking alcohol, 'I became the party girl that I wanted to be, a completely different person.' Staci, on page 161, is the same. 'It was like a switch had been turned on in my head—I felt amazing . . . It made me feel happy and confident and like I was having fun, all the things that I wanted.'

Anna, whose story comes next, on page 175, is also honest about why she went after alcohol so enthusiastically. 'I wanted to be someone who was gregarious and fun, and I couldn't do that naturally. I looked at other people and how comfortable they looked and I wanted to feel that way too.' For many years Anna used alcohol to help her become more comfortable at parties and events. It took quitting drinking completely for her to accept that she's simply not naturally comfortable in crowds. That in actual fact her ideal way to socialise is with small groups of people, and what she finds most energising is spending time alone. Sounds simple, but in a society that appears to favour extraversion, or at least not openly embrace introversion, it's easier said than done.

'I didn't know I was an introvert. I didn't actually even know that introversion was a thing.' That's my friend Sue, reflecting on her early years. 'I knew that I was different from my parents and most other people, because they all seemed like they were having fun, being happy in a group, laughing and joking with each other, doing all this stuff. And I just couldn't keep up. I couldn't meet their energy levels or relate to them.' Like Anna, Sue discovered early on that drinking alcohol gave her confidence in social situations, and helped her not care about how she was really feeling. 'I didn't feel like a misfit when I drank, because I was kind of numb and it maybe dialled down my anxiety a little bit. I'd stop caring about things like whether I fit in or whether I had anything interesting to say. My tongue would definitely loosen up and I would say things that I probably wouldn't have said. I would joke around and maybe flirt more than I normally would have. Alcohol gave me an ability to function socially, something I felt most people could do without help, but I really couldn't.'

I wonder how many people there are like Anna and Sue out there right now, drinking to give themselves confidence and help them fit in. People who believe everyone else around them is being all hunky-dory and super comfortable in social situations, when in reality that's not what's happening at all. Clinical psychologist Karen Nimmo says almost no one feels super confident and has it all worked out. 'We're all struggling with our own sense of self and insecurity. The world is a confusing, tricky place. We're all constantly trying to navigate that and to find our place in it. That can be hard. That's where things like alcohol come in to help us, temporarily at least, feel more comfortable.'

My friend Sue is now in her late fifties and hasn't had a drink for over seven years. After working hard on discovering her true self, she says what's so satisfying now is that she feels very comfortable saying no to social events if she doesn't want to go. 'It is so great, I can't tell you. I feel like I've given myself this huge gift of accepting that I'm totally fine the way I am. Now, if I get invited to something that I know I'm not going to enjoy or want to be part of, I give myself the consideration and the respect of saying, "Thanks for the invitation, but no thank you," and staying home.'

But is it easier to adopt this homebody attitude when you're in your fifties and life has settled down? Sue admits that yes, it probably is. 'When you're younger, the whole socialising thing is really important for finding a mate, having friends, finding friends for your kids, getting promotions at work, being part of the work team. Those were my big drinking years and that was one of the other reasons that I had to drink, to function in that way.'

Single Natalie, newly sober, who told her story on page 138, says dating as a non-drinker can be difficult. 'There is a really significant fear of how you're going to date when you're sober. In my group of female friends, that has been a real concern. It's really hard to be that introverted person and still meet someone. All our cultural rituals around meeting people are around having a drink as well. I think that is actually a really big thing. I think a lot of women have been naturally shy and had a few drinks because they can become the party girl, and then that makes it a bit easier. And then it's a habit that you fall into.'

But, at the end of the day, don't we want a prospective new partner to know and love the real us, insecurities and all, and not some faux, bubbly, tipsy version of ourselves who is desperately trying to appear to be something that we're not? Nimmo tells me a little insecurity can actually be a good thing: 'Self doubt—in small doses—can help you have a reality check around what you're doing, it can help you to correct things that perhaps need correcting, and can just keep you balanced in the way you think about things and your choices.'

Also, don't forget, alcohol is a tricky trickster. It presents itself as a social lubricant, but it's not. And it's not just me saying that. Here's Catharine Fairbairn and Michael Sayette from the University of Pittsburgh's Psychology Department: 'The experimental literature examining alcohol's effects within a social context reveals that alcohol does not consistently enhance social-emotional experience. Alcohol's effects within a social context are largely explained by its tendency to free individuals from preoccupation with social rejection, sedating their limbic and cortical regions, and allowing them to "perceive" social rewards (even if this is not factual).'[1]

You see? Alcohol doesn't consistently enhance our social experiences; it just sedates us, numbs our insecurities and makes us think we're winning socially even when we might not be. It might feel like it's working to give us confidence in the moment, because we're made to feel bubbly and flirty and free, but it's not authentic confidence. It's faux, temporary confidence, not the lovely deep, grounded confidence that comes from knowing, accepting and being who you really are. This real confidence is something many people experience only after they quit drinking.

Here are a few quotes taken from the hundreds of Sober Stories I've published at livingsober.org.nz. Kerry: 'I always thought I was confident, but I had no real idea how much further from the truth that really was. I only thought I was confident because I was drinking. I was so surprised to start feeling positive, confident and HAPPY after I quit. I feel invincible in any situation now.' Michelle: 'I thought it was the normal and harmless thing to do, to grab a drink to feel more confident. Now I'm stronger than I ever thought I could be and realise I didn't need the drink to have confidence.' Ann: 'It was a transformation. Growth into a confident, self-sufficient sober person, with new habits and values.' Gen: 'I gained confidence in myself, belief in my ability to do the things I set out to do.' And Andrea puts it most brilliantly of all: 'Not everyone thinks, feels, lives, acts the same and that's what makes life interesting. Getting sober helped me find myself again. I love being all of me with confidence and genuine respect for who I am. I trust myself, value myself and feel free. That was unfathomable before; now that I have it, I find it's invaluable.'

Now, not everyone needs to quit drinking completely and get sober in order to accept who they are authentically and find their true courage. And not everyone is a through-and-through introvert who is only ever happy spending time with small groups or alone. In actual fact, Nimmo says a lot of people are a bit of both—extraverted in one context and introverted in another—and the goal is to be comfortable with both sides of yourself. That is, being able to be with people socially and also be relaxed when you're on your own, not craving attention or validation from outside sources. But wouldn't it be great if all of us, no matter what our natural social inclination, somehow found the courage to be our authentic selves, rather than feeling the need to drink booze in order to make us feel more sparkly (something I did for many years)?

If we did allow ourselves to be authentically who we are, not only would we feel more grounded and comfortable in our own skin, but we'd also probably find that we'd start to attract the right sort of people to us. People who fit. 'Now that I'm not drinking, and I'm much more of who I am, I attract more people like that,' Sue says. 'Instead of me being at the pub boozing and attracting boozers, I'm actually attracting artists, I'm attracting gardeners—those are the people who I hang out with now. It's like my whole world has realigned and rearranged itself so that I'm now living in a world that I fit. Whereas before I felt like I was jamming myself into something that didn't fit.'

Doesn't living authentically, feeling like you fit and having like-minded people around you sound like the ultimate party? I don't think anyone would require liquid courage to hang out in that space.

26.

Anna

'I looked at other people and how comfortable they looked and I wanted to feel that way too.'

There was alcohol around me growing up, but it wasn't until I became a teenager that it became really widespread. From around thirteen years old I'd go to weddings and older kids would get me a drink. Then from the age of fourteen or fifteen our friends' parents would supply us with alcohol for parties. That was just completely normal and they'd laugh about us: 'Ha ha ha, so-and-so's got a hangover.' We were very young, but it was just a really enabling atmosphere around me. No one was saying, 'Hey, you shouldn't be drinking.' No one talked to me about alcohol and its effects and those kinds of things, I was just like, 'Wow, this makes me feel amazing!' All my anxiety and shyness went away; this was how I wanted to feel.

I was quite a heavy drinker in my teens and into my

twenties. I wouldn't drink at all during the week but then I'd have huge binges on the weekend. There were lots of things I really loved about that. It was fun. I would go out and be loud and dancy and sweary, and I thought that was brilliant. The next day would be rough, but I wanted to be someone who was gregarious and fun and I couldn't do that naturally. I looked at other people and how comfortable they looked and I wanted to feel that way too.

I am the kind of personality that will ruminate and be anxious about almost every conversation that I have. I think, *Did I say something wrong? Do they not like me?* But when I drank I could get rid of those thoughts and feel the way I wanted. I'd feel interesting and funny, but only to a point and then I wasn't fun at all.

It always started well. I'd have just finished work, the sun's shining outside and someone says, 'Let's go and sit in the café and have a glass of wine,' and there was that great feeling of, *I'm with people I like, and I want to drink and I can, and the sun's shining.* That promise of the first wine was just the best thing ever. I would have that first glass and feel like a million bucks. I loved that feeling because it took me out of myself.

I'd convince myself that I could just have one or two, but as soon as I had that first one I knew that I couldn't stop and then it would start to deteriorate. I wasn't being me, I wasn't being authentic, yet I wanted to feel good so badly I would just chase the feeling the rest of the time. I'd get crippling thoughts an hour into the process, so I would then drink a LOT more to try and cover up those feelings.

I always drank too much, but it was sort of okay. The

functional alcoholic thing, that wasn't a discussion. There were alcoholics, but they were people who slept in the park or stayed at home and drank. I would run my drinking through my own filter of what I thought an alcoholic was and think, *No, you're okay, because you don't drink in the morning and you don't drink all day.*

Then my marriage broke up and I went from drinking maybe three nights a week to daily, and to a dangerous degree. I had rules for myself: only drink a bottle, don't open that second bottle, that sort of thing. But you know, you break your rules: *Oh, I'll just have one glass out of the second bottle*, and then it's gone. I would have conversations with myself when I drove home: *No not today, you don't need it*, and then at the last possible supermarket I'd always stop and tell myself, *Well if I don't drink it tonight I'll have it tomorrow.*

If I ever went to work drinks I'd only stay for a short time, 'cause I knew if I stayed too long I'd get drunk and make a fool of myself. So I'd go for an hour—it'd be the golden hour to feel amazing. By the time I got in the car I'd be like, *Shit, I really need another drink*, so I'd buy something on the way home, get home and get plastered. Then knowing I had to get to work the next day, I'd find myself sitting in the shower crying and crying, not wanting to live anymore. That was the cycle. The following night: *Woah, I feel bad about myself. A drink would take the edge off that.* You know the story. The things that it promises it does deliver, but for such a short moment in time and then it makes everything worse. Everything.

I took my drinking indoors because I realised that I was

making a fool of myself going to work drinks and stuff, so I pulled it right back so that all my drinking pretty much was done at home. I'd bulldoze my children into their beds and do the quickest story-time ever and breathe wine fumes all over them, and then get out so I could get back to my glass of wine. I almost had that deadline for myself. I might have had one after I got home after work but I'd really get stuck in after they got into bed. I was always pissed from seven o'clock onwards.

I was just doing my best with the stuff that was going on, and I can always look back and think, *Well, my husband had an affair and he left, and then this happened and this happened—it's no wonder I was in a state.* But the drinking was there so I couldn't see that. I actually tried lots and lots of times to do something about it. I went and had counselling once, which was helpful, but the counsellor actually said to me at one point that my drinking was at the low end of the scale and perhaps I could just cut down.

People around me said, 'We all have a lot to drink.' I was reaching out but not really able to grasp on to someone who said, 'Yeah you have got a problem.' In the end it was a personal realisation that I was smashing myself over the head with a brick. *You can't be happy if you drink, so just stop.* And it finally came down to that. *You can't have both. You can't be happy and drink alcohol so one's got to go. Which one is it?*

I'm really proud of what I've done, but I haven't yet been able to completely move on from the fact that I was having a shocker. I still feel shame; I haven't done anything with that. When I really started to drink heavily I never matured or grew up so it wasn't just the drinking. I wasn't doing the things I needed to, to really cope with my life. Financially, emotionally. I was functioning in terms of having good jobs and parenting, but definitely not parenting to the best of my ability. I was a real mess. For a long time I felt all on my own with the whole thing.

I haven't had a drink for over nine years now, and I'm still finding out who I am. Who is the person who doesn't drink, and how am I entertaining or fun to be around? I don't drink anymore, but it's not a magic bullet. There's other stuff I've got to do to be okay.

I'm hopeless at getting together with people. In a horrible sort of admission, I realise now that a huge part of going out was just because I wanted to drink, not because I wanted to have quality conversations with people. I had a recent experience at work where they held a training evening and we had to go and learn a new system in the office. And I thought, *Uh-oh*. And the first thing that happened when I walked in was I was offered a glass of wine. I always hesitate to say 'I don't drink' in those situations because I think it's going to make other people feel uncomfortable, particularly with women. I think they'll either not want to be friends with me or the conversation will falter because it's awkward. People almost treat it like you've just said you're sick or somebody died. Sometimes I make jokes about it. If somebody says, 'Oh, why don't you drink?' I'll make a joke and say, 'Well, I was way too good at drinking.' In a way sometimes I think that's almost glorifying it as well, but it's easier to do than have that silence.

I now know I get my energy from being on my own, and I love spending time with people in small groups. So before

I was just being someone who I wasn't and that might have been part of why drinking made me so anxious. Because, actually, the drug was making me live outside of who I really was and what I was comfortable with. Now, finally, I am realising that. And being sober for me is the greatest thing. Yes, I still have things to deal with—but we all do. Every day I am grateful to be living without drink. I can't imagine ever going back to it. It lurks there, but life is so much better now that I'm not interested.

27.

The Superwoman problem

It may well be that the reason so many women drink alcohol at the end of the day is because we're bone tired. We're tired, stressed and strung out from doing a million things all day, for the umpteenth day in a row. We're tired, stressed and strung out from working hard at our jobs, keeping our homes tidy and organised, caring for our partners, parenting our kids, keeping the pets and/or houseplants alive, being reliable friends and daughters and workmates and neighbours, maintaining our nails and eyebrows and teeth, refraining from eating too much sugar and gluten and dairy and meat, avoiding single-use plastic and chemical toxins and bugs, keeping up with the latest news and podcasts and literature, practising mindfulness and yoga, staying fashionable and up to date with the latest trends in makeup and hair, and . . . the list goes on. I'm exhausted just typing it all out.

We're doing it all, all the time, and it's bloody exhausting.

Even though we may be, on the surface at least, managing to mostly keep it all together and perform our tasks adequately, inside we're likely dying a slow death from the sheer effort of it all. I actually just got the giggles while I typed that sentence, because here I am writing a chapter on how women are run ragged from doing so much and I'm currently sitting at the library on a public holiday, working hard, necking pain killers and cough mixture because I've got a head cold, feeling exhausted because I slept badly and got up early to tidy the kitchen and put a load of washing on before coming here to work all day. Knowing that, from here, I'm heading straight to the airport to pick up my son, and after we get home I need to put clean sheets on his bed and his brother's and answer some overdue emails. I am the embodiment of the woman trying to do it all (work, parent, run a house, stay well), and I'm only just managing to hold myself together. I'm trying to be Superwoman, and it's a problem.

Debora Spar, author of the book *Wonder Women: Sex, power, and the quest for perfection*, says the Superwoman myth grew out of feminism in the 1970s and was fed to us through images on TV. 'If you look at the images of professional women that started to emerge in the 1970s, and that are still out there today, the good news is that we see women being cops and surgeons and detectives and all of these very intriguing careers, the bad news is that we see these women still looking like models, managing to have husbands and children without ever really getting frustrated by that combination of things. If young women are constantly being pummelled by these images, not only on television but also in movies, magazine stands, they start to set their expectations higher and higher. So that they begin to feel that if they're not running the corporate law firm and putting the perfect dinner on the table and keeping the perfect home and being totally sexy all of the time, that they're somehow falling short.'[1]

We feel like we're falling short if we don't pull off the endless juggle of roles and expectations with ease. We feel like we're falling short if we snap at our kids while standing at the kitchen bench shovelling mini bags of chips into our mouth. We feel like we're falling short if we cry in the toilets at work because our boss is being difficult and we were awake at 3 a.m. worrying about our relationship. We feel like we're falling short, and on top of that we feel guilty.

Jess Stuart is an author, motivational speaker and coach who makes a living out of helping women deal with the stresses and pressures of modern life. She told me guilt is one of the biggest issues women face when trying to do it all. 'We've got equal opportunity, so that's great because now you get to smash the glass ceiling as well as be an awesome mother. But then women get themselves to this point where they want to be doing well at work yet they're having to miss meetings because they also want to pick up their kids from school. Or they're staying late to work and now they feel guilty for not being at the school games. So it's that constant feeling of guilt because they're juggling all the balls. And at one part, something's kind of falling away because we can't keep it all perfect.'

This guilt and feeling of falling short is affecting women right across the board, as Spar says: 'Women across the socioeconomic spectrum are feeling the same problems of frustration, of expectations and sadly of guilt and of failure. These are problems that really cut across. Women feel guilty regardless of where they work and how much they make and how many kids they have. That seems to be a proverbial problem right now, and that's one that I really think we need to tackle.'[2]

We do need to tackle it. But how? For many of us we tackle it in the easiest, cheapest, fastest way we know how: by drinking alcohol. We reach for that readily available, cheap-as-chips, glorified liquid hailed left, right and centre as being the golden ticket to relaxation. The drink we've been conditioned to believe from a very young age is the perfect 'treat' or 'reward' that we 'deserve' for all our hard work. Alcohol. And it works. In the short term anyway, it works. It hits our bodies and brains, slows down the central nervous system and produces feel-good chemicals in our brains. It calms us down, relaxes our bodies, silences our busy minds. Sweet relief. As Charmaine says in her story, coming up next on page 187, 'The drinking was just a release from life, a release from responsibility, more than anything else.'

Stuart, who has talked to thousands of women at workshops, events, retreats and during one-on-one coaching sessions, says most women believe alcohol is a good way to fix the feelings of stress, guilt and overwhelm, despite the often negative impacts. 'It's interesting because it makes you feel worse but it's a socially acceptable solution. Women will often joke with their colleagues that they've been trying to have two wine-free days a week but it's gone down to one because their job is so stressful or their life is so busy. It's almost the accepted coping mechanism that they feel they can talk about. If they were saying that they'd had to turn to antidepressants or anti-anxiety meds for the same coping mechanisms they wouldn't talk about it in the same way.'

The problem, of course, with using alcohol as a coping mechanism is that the release is temporary and does nothing to address the actual problems—the mounting pressures and endless responsibilities. Tasks haven't been lessened, demands haven't eased, needy kids are still there, the bulging inbox is still there, the tricky colleagues are still there, the endless piles of washing are still there, the health worries are still there, the worries about the state of the world are still there. The frustrations, expectations and guilt are still there. It's all still there. Except now there may be an extra layer of guilt on top of it all, which is guilt about our drinking.

'In that moment, you feel like the edge has been taken off, you feel your shoulders relax and you're like, *Yes!*' says Stuart. 'But then often you wake up with a hangover and you're not as good as you should be at doing all of the house chores or anything else you've got lined up. I think that's when we get that sense of guilt kick in. Guilt for not being a good mum because you couldn't get up bright and breezy. Guilt as well that you didn't look after yourself properly. Maybe you're supposed to be on a diet yet you had that extra bottle of wine. Another reason to beat ourselves up.'

Stuart works with women to help them find effective, long-term ways to take the pressure off, including replacing drinking with healthier, more nourishing habits. And for those who love to have a glass of wine with friends to unwind? 'If you try and unpick what it is that you love about that,' she says, 'it's generally not the wine. It's generally the social connection, so start another ritual around that.' And finally, she says, take a good look at your to-do list. Is everything you've got on your plate really a priority? 'If we could only pick five things off that list to do, and we picked out the real priorities, we'd find that the rest of the stuff wasn't actually that urgent. When we take things off the list, when we slow down and take time out, what we actually find is that that helps us speed up because we become more effective. It doesn't take as long for us to do that stuff because we're a bit sharper, more focused and more grounded. I try and help women see that, by shortening their to-do lists and taking time out, they'll actually do more and they'll be more effective at what they do.'

So if you're run ragged, at the end of your tether, with a groaning to-do list and a gnawing sense of falling short and guilt, ask yourself: What do I really need to do right now to help me with this situation? For me right now, as I sit coughing and spluttering at the library with a heavy head and a huge to-do list, it's not going home and downing a bottle of merlot like I would have eight or so years ago. It's going home and putting my comfy pants on, lying on the sofa and watching some mindless TV. It's having a mug of chamomile tea, not emptying my inbox but maybe emailing my publisher to say that I need an extension on delivering my manuscript. All the while feeling okay about taking the pressure off, because even though I'm a hard-working superstar I'm not Superwoman, and nor do I want to be.

28.

Charmaine

'The drinking was just a release from life, a release from responsibility.'

I grew up in an environment where there was a lot of drinking going on. We lived in a little village where people socialised together a lot. I saw drinking as a happy and fun thing to do, but I did have an awareness of it having a dark side, because my grandmother was a closet alcoholic. My father was a drinker; he was a fun, sociable person. My mother didn't drink much at all—she was at home looking after us, probably not having much fun at all.

I didn't drink at all as a teenager; I didn't like it. I started when I found myself as a single mother in my early twenties. My husband and I separated and I was left with our four-month-old baby, and I started meeting with friends to socialise. We used to sit around with our children and drink casks of wine—it felt safe but we were drinking way too much. It was always to excess and inevitably I'd get sick. But it was fun. I don't remember using alcohol to deal with emotion; it was more like 'Friday night, let your hair down' stuff.

When I think back it was when wine went into the supermarkets, that's when things got worse. Every week, bottles went in my trolley; it was just natural, a habit. I wouldn't drink every day during the week at home. If I did, mostly it was just a glass or two. I'm a teacher and you can't teach with a hangover, it's just horrendous. So I held it together during the week, and then I'd hit the weekend like, *Yippee, it's Friday, let my hair down! I can do this now, and I'm gonna go for it.* I became the party girl that I wanted to be, a completely different person. I'm probably a bit lacking in confidence in that sense. It gave me false confidence. The problem was I couldn't control it. I would go with every intention of having one or two glasses, and then have one or two bottles. I don't have a switch that says 'stop, that's enough'. So when other people go, *Oh, I had a few wines. I don't think I'll have any more*, I just keep on going until I'm vomiting.

I remarried, and the norm within our group of friends—middle-class, white, rural people—was to drink to excess. And over time it got really hideous. I got to the stage that whenever I drank I couldn't remember a lot of the night. I would have memory blanks every time, then wake up embarrassed, with terrible guilt, and ask people, 'What was I doing?' They'd say, 'I couldn't even notice any difference. You just behaved normally.' I knew it was wrong that I couldn't remember, but other people didn't seem to think it was. Anything could have happened to me. Absolutely anything and I wouldn't have had a clue.

I also drove drunk a few times, putting my life and the lives of other people on the roads at risk. One night I drove 30 kilometres home and woke up in the morning with no recollection of getting there at all. I thought, *Oh my god, I'm going to kill someone. If I keep doing this I could lose my husband, my career and the wonderful life I have.* That was the last time I ever had a drink.

The thing for me that I found so hard, going back nine years now since I quit, was that I felt really alone in what I was doing. Not drinking wasn't out there in the public at all, and every single person I knew drank. The only person I found who didn't drink smoked so much dope it wasn't funny, so that wasn't any help. I tried AA for a while, and they were lovely people but I didn't feel like I fitted in. In the end I thought, *I'm the higher power here. I can control this. I can make the choice not to drink again*, which I did.

One of the best things I did when I gave up was to go to a gym and tell them exactly what was going on. It was a little privately owned gym and they were lovely. So I got quite fit and I think the endorphins made me feel good about myself and my body. I started running and I'd never been a runner before. I did a couple of half-marathons when I was 45, and I think it just gave me a sense of purpose. I'd always run at about five o'clock at night, and I think it gave me those same feelings that a glass of wine had given me.

I also had counselling, which was great. She was very good, because she'd been an alcoholic herself. At first I just tried cutting down and she said to me, 'If you stop and you start again, you won't go back gradually, you'll be instantly back to where you were.' And I thought, *Well I can't ever go back then, because I was at the stage where I was going to lose everything if I carried on.* She also told me, 'You will end up like your grandmother,' which was quite a sobering thought. She asked me, 'What is it that you like about it?' I said, 'It's fitting in with a group of girlfriends, having lunch with a nice wine or whatever.' She then said to me, 'You can still socialise. What about if you had something else in your glass?' So I carried on doing things, and I always have a wine glass, but with lemon lime and bitters in it or whatever. I've found what I actually like is the situation, being around people and friends and socialising, that sort of thing.

My counsellor also helped me establish that I'd always been a super-responsible person. My mum was only eighteen when she had me, then when I was three my twin brothers were born and right from the word go I helped out with them. After having a planned baby at 21, my then-husband left me when the baby was only a few months old, so I was solely responsible for my own child from the age of 21. And I've always worked as a teacher, so I've always had these responsible roles. The drinking was just a release from life, a release from responsibility, more than anything else.

It was hard for a while after I quit because my husband carried on drinking socially. He knew I was going to counselling and stuff, but I don't think he believed that I could do it. It's not that he didn't support me, but I had to prove to him that I could do it. Now he's so supportive and has pulled himself back a bit from the drinking too. Nine years down the track and we're very, very happy. We've got lovely kids and I'm a principal now.

Five o'clock comes and goes and I don't think about it to be honest—I've broken the habit now.

I can see the positives now in what I did, that I actually turned it around. It was massive and I'm really proud of it. We need to get the message out more that you can have a really fulfilled life and be really happy without touching alcohol at all.

29.
Self-medicating

For me, giving up alcohol was a fairly straightforward process. I'm not saying it was easy, but it was straightforward. I reached my point of change (hard, painful), made the decision to quit (scary, exciting), learned how to live without drinking (complex, eye-opening) and developed new coping mechanisms (drawn-out, rewarding). Jeepers, I have never summarised my recovery journey in such a concise way! Of course there's so much more that went into it than this, and I have written two memoirs (*Mrs D is Going Without* and *Mrs D is Going Within*) that go through all of it in great detail, but in short this is what I did. I removed alcohol and learned how to beat cravings, socialise sober, shift hardwired thoughts around booze, sit with uncomfortable emotions and manage mood fluctuations. Again, summarising massively but this gives you the bare bones. It wasn't a walk in the park by any means, but it was fairly bog standard as far as recovery journeys go.

For some people, this is not the way it goes. For some people, removing alcohol leads to a far more complex process.

They take the alcohol away and find that underneath there are some pretty major mental or physical issues (or both) that require serious work. 'Getting sober is often considered the ultimate solution to our problems,' writes author, coach and founder of livsrecoverykitchen.com, Olivia Pennelle, on The Fix, 'And in many ways, it is. We stop the behaviors that led to the self-destruction to our bodies, our relationships, and how we live our lives. We wake up without feeling hungover or in withdrawal from drugs we'd taken the night before. By dealing with the issues that led to using, we begin to experience healing and generally feel better. But for some of us, that isn't enough. Physically, we can actually feel worse after we stop using or drinking. We may discover that drugs and alcohol were masking the symptoms of a serious and deeply rooted illness.'[1]

She's speaking from experience. Shortly after entering recovery, Pennelle was hit with debilitating chronic fatigue, which eventually led to the diagnosis of an autoimmune disease and complex PTSD from a series of traumas throughout her lifetime. 'Once I removed the drug, I removed the anesthesia. I was so desperate. I was so broken. I was so raw. It was very challenging to function,' she says. Figuring out what was going on was a long and arduous process that involved much confusion, misdiagnoses, frustration and pain.

My friend Michelle found herself going through an equally difficult and gruelling process after she quit. She thought going booze-free would make her feel like a million bucks, but instead she spent most of her days feeling like she had been run over by a bulldozer. 'I felt ripped off. I had stopped drinking and got this?' She had terrible pain in her joints, hot flushes, anxiety, depression and brain fog. After a couple of years, many visits to a specialist and trials of different medicines, she was diagnosed with fibromyalgia—a complex condition involving bones, muscles and a lot of pain. 'No alcohol in my system uncovered a load of things. The fibromyalgia was one, but I also discovered that menopause was raising its ugly head, which fibro magnifies the symptoms of.'

Another friend of mine, Matt, fell into an extremely dark place after he stopped his regular drinking habit. The two years following his last drink were a rollercoaster of anxiety, panic attacks and a major depressive episode that led to a breakdown. 'I had long suffered from down times, and in hindsight I can see that I probably always dealt with anxiety. But I'd never really dealt with my problems properly when I drank. Avoidance and hiding away was my main tool, and alcohol was the perfect drug to take the edge off uncomfortable feelings. Without alcohol I felt the anxiety in a far more physical way and my depression was far more raw.'

Louise, whose story features later in the book, on page 255, had a similar experience after putting the drink down. 'I felt awful for the first six months. I was emotionally fragile and battling big time with massive untreated depression and anxiety. I was also perimenopausal and had a lot of pain in my back . . . It took a few years to sort myself out. I had a lot of medical help and wonderful recovery folk helping me to separate my alcoholism from other conditions.'

Cases like these are far from uncommon. Here in New Zealand statistics show that at least 70 per cent of people who attend alcohol and drug services are likely to have coexisting mental-health disorders.[2] In Australia, studies show that women with general anxiety disorders and social anxiety are more likely to misuse alcohol.[3]

There's an awful lot to unpick and discuss when it comes to mental health, diseases and coexisting conditions—far more than I could ever do in great depth here—but what I can say is that having a lot of alcohol in the mix can make it very difficult to properly identify, let alone address and treat, many issues. Take the alcohol away, however, or at least drastically reduce it, like Rebecca who shares her story next, on page 198, and things become much clearer and easier to deal with. As many people have discovered, the extra effort it takes to drill down into underlying issues is well worth it.

Nowadays Olivia Pennelle takes care of her physical and mental well-being with trauma-focused psychotherapy, regular exercise, sufficient sleep, outdoor activities, community and alternative medicine. She advocates for her needs with doctors and seeks referrals to specialists when necessary. 'It's about building my self-esteem but also learning coping strategies through therapy—that's been one of the most profound supports that I've sought. Because you don't necessarily know those coping skills when you have substance use disorder and/ or complex PTSD. I didn't. It's a relief to finally be figuring myself out.'

Michelle changed her diet and addressed the symptoms of her menopause, both of which helped with the fibromyalgia. But there was still more work to be done. 'I realised my mind and body needed a better connection. They'd been dancing to a different tune for years while I numbed them out with booze and I'd never really given them the chance to live in sync. So now I work hard to try and feel and understand what my body is telling me, and cut my stress off at the pass before it has a chance to travel to my body. It's a huge work in progress but I'm enjoying my life so much more now. I've dealt with this health issue with strength I wouldn't have had if I was still drinking.'

Louise says sorting out her underlying issues took 'a lot of love, sleep, patience, discipline and rigorous honesty to get through each day, and recover my life one step at a time'. She now takes hormone-replacement therapy for some of the symptoms of perimenopause, and has had psychiatric help for depression and anxiety. 'The back pain I'm just managing with Panadol and ibuprofen. The result is peace, health and sobriety, and it's priceless. It's life itself.'

As for Matt, he's now doing so well he's written a book charting his mental-health journey. In *The Longest Day: Standing up to depression and tackling the Coast to Coast* he discusses all of the tools he's developed to keep himself well. Things like exercise, yoga, mindfulness and gratitude. Resting when needed, taking medication every morning and checking in with his counsellor when the balance goes out. 'I'm a far more content and connected person. It's a day-to day thing still, but things are far more even and I'm more aware of the signs of slipping back into severe depression.'

One of the biggest tools in Matt's toolbox is fostering friendships and connections with others who understand what he's going through. 'The emotional rollercoaster I found myself on was made all the easier, or maybe less surprising, because I was connected to the experience of others at livingsober.org.nz, many of whom also had mental-health issues rise up after they quit. When you're reading blogs and hearing consistent messages about "living in the raw" and having to be brave and face the world and yourself without booze, it softens the experience. I never went back to drinking because I knew it wouldn't help. It would have been like pouring petrol on to a forest fire.'

30.

Rebecca

'I was actually probably quite high in terms of my mental health at times.'

I come from a stereotypical white, middle-class family. I have clear memories of Mum and Dad stocking up on a monthly supply of booze from the local neighbourhood liquor store on the company charge account. A big trolley full of casks of Müller-Thurgau and Country—those wines everyone drank back in the 1980s. They had a really big group of friends and were very social, lots of fancy-dress parties. Drinking was normalised, it was part of the social milieu as a family, and I presumed that's just the way it happens. People would have dinner parties and parents got a bit funny and danced and you didn't think anything different.

I probably had the odd sip of alcohol at a barbecue when I was about fifteen or something, but not much. Around the sixteen-year-old mark, that's when I started going to parties where alcohol was a big feature. You wouldn't go to a party without getting some booze. We started going to nightclubs with fake ID, dancing and looking all grown-up with our makeup and big hair, just getting completely boozed. Sometimes we'd go down to the park on a Friday night and get a four-pack of Miami wine coolers and that would last us the weekend.

I was quite a high achiever when I was younger, but then I started having self-esteem issues and my relationship with my mother became a bit strained. I was having a bit of a gritty time, trying to find my way. I started at university and the drinking got pretty crazy. We had this drinking game where we'd split into three or four different teams and each team would swallow a different colour of food colouring, so you'd know who'd spewed. First team to spew lost. I mean that's foul, fucking disgusting. We're talking eighteen-year-olds.

Throughout that first year of uni, that's when things took a stage dive. My marks plummeted, my parents' marriage broke up, and I think this is when the depression came on. But I didn't know that. I was trying to navigate all this stuff while having these really core mental-health issues, but not really recognising what it was. I went down to Queenstown and worked for a season. I thought something was wrong with my environment, not me. I think I was running away. I was twenty, working two or three jobs, training, drinking heaps, lots of risky sexual behaviour, everything. I'd get boozed, go to some guy's house, then wake up and think, *Fuck, what have I done?* and grab a taxi home. Pretty quickly

I collapsed—mentally and physically. I got admitted to Queenstown hospital, where they said it was depression and that I'd had a hypomanic episode. That was probably the first moment that a doctor diagnosed a mental-health issue. I was on hospital bed rest for about four or five days and then got back to it and continued on with the same sort of behaviour.

I moved back to Christchurch and studied for another year, but ended up pulling out of university and moving again, this time up to Auckland. I was still quite heavily binge drinking. I'd have periods when I'd wake up and go, *Fuck, I must have blacked out. I can't remember bits from that night.* I'd have to get a girlfriend to fill me in on the details. We all did; it wasn't uncommon.

I was starting to beat myself up about the drinking through my twenties. I'd say to myself, 'I'm not going to drink again,' but then Friday night would roll around. I would never, ever think about going to a party or out to a bar or anything without drinking. It made me pretty vulnerable as I'd go wandering off by myself. It'd be late at night and I'd get sick of my friends, so I'd go off and cruise around K' Road by myself. I once went back to a guy's house and it could have led to rape, but I managed to pull myself away. Looking back now I was lucky that nothing really bad happened.

I was feeling lost and absolutely, totally shaky. I didn't know where I fitted in. Through my whole childhood I'd been this high achiever, on the school council, getting arts awards, speech and drama awards—it had given me a sense of achievement. Maybe it was a semi ego trip, but it was where I got recognition, especially from my family. Then when things fell off the jetty a bit in my late teens and twenties and I pulled out of university, I felt lost in myself and was seeking a place of belonging. I made some really good friends in Auckland, but I was still an outsider living in a big city with no sense of place. I thought by that time of life I would have graduated and be an account manager at Saatchi & Saatchi or something. I had part-time jobs but not career jobs. God forbid if I'd ever bumped into anyone I knew from school. At least when I was drinking I felt okay.

I can remember being really unwell with depression, lying in bed during the day and wishing the hours would hurry up and tick on until the evening. Because at least by then everyone else who was working would be at home or out socialising, and we're all the same in the evening. We're all out and about having this fabulous time, and that's when I felt like I belonged. I got my sense of belonging with partying and alcohol.

I met my partner in my mid twenties, and we made quite a team. He levelled me out. It's funny—in retrospect I was actually probably quite high in terms of my mental health at times, but not knowing what that meant. So when I was totally animated I'd be like, 'Come on! Let's go do this or that!' and he'd say, 'Come on, babe, chill out. Let's do this.' He'd be more relaxed and I would try to pep him up. We were together for ten years, and during that time I had a bit more security. I still had really full-on bouts of depression though.

We split up and a while after that I went back to see my GP. I was really unwell with depression and we talked about how I'd been hospitalised a couple of times. She said, 'I think you might have bipolar.' I was then put into an eighteen-month bipolar study. The hypothesis they were trying to prove was that taking medication and having regular talking therapy as well as being monitored by a psychiatrist would lead to a better long-term outcome than just seeing your GP. I was put on lithium and the fog lifted. I could manage the highs and lows a bit better. I've been well ever since then, but I have kept on drinking. About four years ago I lost my driver's licence. I'd been drinking over four or five hours, I think I'd had about five glasses of wine, and I hadn't had anything to eat. So that was a pretty low point, going to court. I have to disclose that on any job application now.

About two years ago I thought my drinking was getting a bit heavy. I was probably up to about four bottles of wine a week, and I thought, *Fuck, I actually need to unpeel this and get to the crux of the issue.* I knew it wasn't a major issue like it used to be, but I could see down the vortex so I went and had some sessions with a counsellor. She had me keep an alcohol log, which we'd go over, and we'd also plan ahead. She was good and I cut right back. I've now got a saying that I came up with: 'Wine is for sharing', which means it's only to be enjoyed when I'm with company. I don't keep wine in the house, just in case. I just did Dry July because I saw it as a good chance to draw a line in the sand and make a concerted effort to put health and well-being at the forefront. I actually started in mid June to get a head start. I have a SodaStream machine, so soda and lemon is my drink of choice—in a nice glass, of course. I'm noticing how clear my thoughts are in the mornings and how my skin is glowing. I am going away next weekend, but I am conscious of making good, controlled choices. It's not an easy relationship that I have with alcohol, but I'm conscious of it. It's a work in progress.

31.

Adverse Childhood Experiences

One final word about what might be behind people's drinking before I move on to the final part of the book, in which I'll discuss changing habits and living without a crap-tonne of alcohol in your life (my favourite topic!). Here I just want to touch on some powerful and compelling research that has been carried out around the world looking at the long-term impacts from trauma during childhood.

The research is called the Adverse Childhood Experiences Study (or ACE Study),[1] and it looks at the impact of childhood trauma on a person's life. It was first carried out in the United States in the mid 1990s, and has since been replicated in many other places, including New Zealand.[2] Tens of thousands of individuals have taken part. What the ACE Study does is look for traumatic events (they call them 'Adverse Childhood Experiences' or ACEs for short) that happened in a person's life when they were young, and then for the physical and emotional health outcomes that subsequently occurred for them later in life. The findings are clear: the more trauma you experienced in your childhood, the more likely you are to have ongoing health impacts later in your life.

'The Adverse Childhood Experiences Study is something that everybody needs to know about,' says Nadine Burke Harris in her TED Talk 'How childhood trauma affects health across a lifetime'.[3] She's a paediatrician and has just been appointed as the first ever Surgeon General of California. 'We now understand better than we ever have before how exposure to early adversity affects the brains and bodies of children.'

The ACE Study looks at ten types of childhood traumas: physical abuse, emotional abuse, sexual abuse, physical neglect, emotional neglect, mental illness in the home, substance abuse in the home, mother treated violently, divorce, and having an incarcerated relative. For each ACE experienced you get a score of 1, so if you have three of those traumas present in your childhood, your score is 3. The negative health impacts in later life that are recorded are things like smoking, intravenous drug use, heart disease, HIV, depression, suicidality, and alcohol use disorder.

Just a quick note about 'alcohol use disorder', because it's one of those terms that's used in the clinical world but not by the rest of us in everyday conversations. Alcohol use disorder covers a wide-ranging spectrum, from what we'd probably call 'drinking issues' at the mild end to 'alcoholism' at the severe end. Signs of an alcohol use disorder are things like having problems controlling alcohol intake, thinking about alcohol all the time, continuing to drink even when it causes problems, having to drink more to get the same effect, and having withdrawal symptoms.

According to the ACE Study, if you've had no childhood trauma and your ACE score is 0, your chances of having an alcohol use disorder are quite low—one in 69. Your chances jump massively to one in nine if you've got a score of 1–3. A score of 7 or more ACEs and your chance is even higher— one in six. Put simply: there's a proven reason why so many of us drink to levels that aren't good for us, and, as clichéd as it sounds, it can be clearly traced back to childhood. As one of the ACE Study's authors, Vincent J. Felitti, puts it, for many of us our problem drinking is a 'readily understandable although largely unconscious attempt to gain relief from well-concealed prior life traumas by using psychoactive materials'.[4] These prior life traumas are well-concealed, he says, because of shame, secrecy and social taboo. And the reason attempts to gain relief are largely unconscious is because people with ACEs have literally had their hardwiring altered.

As Burke Harris spells out in her TED Talk, childhood trauma fundamentally changes the way we are built. If we experience trauma when we're young, it changes how our prefrontal cortex develops (needed for impulse control and executive function), the way our amygdala develops (the brain's fear and response centre), and also 'areas like the nucleus accumbens, the pleasure and reward centre of the brain that is implicated in substance dependence'. It's no mystery—it's science.

Author and coach Olivia Pennelle says it's vital we become more trauma-aware when looking to resolve addiction issues or substance use disorders. She's passionate about raising awareness of the impacts of childhood trauma, having unpicked her own history after she entered recovery. 'I had a very stressful childhood growing up in a household with substance misuse. I relocated to the UK at just three years old and started a new life in a single-parent family. I didn't have the emotional support and attention that I needed, I suffered terribly from my father's abandonment, and consequently I developed maladaptive coping strategies: eating disorders, smoking, and addiction. Through nearly two years of therapy and by doing intensive research—including into the ACE Study—I now understand the strong psychological link between my childhood and my sickness.'[5]

Pennelle believes it's critical we remain open to exploring the impacts of our childhoods on our adult lives. 'If you don't deal with it, then once you remove the substances it's going to be too incredibly painful. We just need to be conscious that if there is any kind of trauma there, you might require professional assistance.'

As difficult as it might seem, facing up to and addressing the deep pain that lingers from childhood trauma is the only way to properly manage it. Squashing it down with alcohol and other things, while an understandable action to take, is misguided—a temporary solution to a permanent problem.

'Pain is unrelenting. It will get our attention,' researcher and storyteller Brené Brown says in her book *Braving the Wilderness: The quest for true belonging and the courage to stand alone*.[6] 'Despite our attempts to drown it in addiction, to physically beat it out of one another, to suffocate it with success and material trappings, or to strangle it with our hate, pain will find a way to make itself known. Pain will subside only when we acknowledge it and care for it. Addressing it with love and compassion would take only a minuscule percentage of the energy it takes to fight it. When we deny our emotion, it owns us. When we own our emotion, we can rebuild and find our way through the pain.'

32.

Jackie

*'Sometimes I wonder how things would be
different if the abuse never happened.'*

I loved it when Mum and Dad drank, as strange as that
sounds, because they worked hard and were very stressed
a lot of the time. They were so busy I didn't really feel like
they had all that much time for us, but when they drank they
became completely different—laid-back and relaxed enough
to muck around with us. When they had a party, it would
be huge and I thought it was the best thing ever. I'd get out
of bed and try and watch them—they'd all be singing and
having a ball and I couldn't wait to get old enough to be able
to do this. It looked so awesome.

My start with alcohol wasn't great. I was given it aged
twelve by a next-door neighbour. He'd just moved in, and
because Mum and Dad had such an active social life they
were like, 'Oh great—a babysitter!' So they'd go out and we

would stay there. But he was awful. He ended up sexually abusing me. It was horrible and ongoing, and I didn't say anything about it for a very long time because I didn't want Mum and Dad to know.

I had always been a really good little girl, good at school, never causing any trouble, but after the abuse started I changed. I started smoking, drinking, acting out and stuff. I remember one New Year's Eve party, I must have been about fourteen, a friend and I started sneaking people's glasses off the tables and drinking them. That was the first time I got really drunk on my own and it was amazing. My friend ended up throwing up, but I just kept on talking away, thinking it was great fun. I had confidence for the first time.

When I was fifteen I finally said something about the abuse to a teacher, thinking it would just be between us, but it all blew up and we ended up going to the social services. It went to court, but I didn't take it any further because it was awful feeling like I was on trial.

By seventeen I was drinking as much as I could, just always binging. If I could go out on Wednesday night, I would, then Thursday night is 'dollar drink' night, and then, of course, Friday, Saturday nights were big, and there was always a Sunday session. I was drinking massive amounts, as much as I could. I remember being afraid, almost terrified that I wouldn't be able to drink enough to get drunk. So I'd get somewhere and order a few drinks really quickly, just to make sure that I got that feeling of being drunk and numb and confident. The big, number-one thing was confidence, 'cause I just didn't have it. On top of the abuse, I'd been bullied at primary school quite badly, so I think I just had issues with confidence. Alcohol was my answer to that.

When I have the urge to drink, it's so powerful. It's like a switch is flicked and it's very hard to argue with that switch. It's almost like I have no control, like I'm being driven by something else all of a sudden, something bigger than me. As soon as I make the decision to drink it's like a chemical reaction. My whole state changes and I go into a state of excitement. The weight of the world comes off my shoulders and all of a sudden I'm happy and carefree. The problem is I can never have just a couple of glasses; once I start I don't want to stop.

Around twenty I started to realise that I had a choice to make. I was hanging around with a group of older musicians, partying hard. It was heaps of fun, but after one weekend full of drugs and alcohol I had a bit of an epiphany. I could see things going downhill fast, so I pulled back after that to just weekend drinking. I've been responsible ever since, working hard in good jobs, but I've kept on having at least two huge party nights pretty much every weekend. If I look at it, basically since I was fourteen or fifteen I've been pretty much drinking every weekend.

When I was in my mid twenties Mum and Dad bought a pub in a beautiful coastal town, and asked me to move up there with them to run it. I did that for eight years and loved it, but pub life is pretty conducive to drinking. It wasn't uncommon for me to have three big binges in a week, and there were times when I was only just keeping myself together. I knew it was a problem and went through some periods of sobriety, even went to AA for some time.

Last year I did a hundred days off and that was huge—

the most I've ever done in my life. I started off really positively and looking back now it was awesome, but there were struggles. Socially it was awkward at times because I've always leaned on alcohol for confidence, but mainly I felt like I was letting people down by not drinking. People were so disappointed, postponing events until I was due to start drinking again. I had friends saying, 'Can't you just drink with me tonight and then start again tomorrow?'

Maybe the problem is I'm very friendly when I'm drinking, hugging and kissing people and having fun. Maybe if my drinking was negative, if I was a fighter or whatever, then people would understand. But right now they don't see it as a problem. They don't understand how embarrassed I get when I overdo it and fall over or vomit. They don't see me depressed in bed for two days after a big bender. They don't see the come-down.

I also have to put up with so much shit from my family when I take a break. They're all big drinkers and when I stop they give me hell. They're like, 'Come on, why aren't you drinking? We're not going to talk to you if you're not drinking.' It's like being an outcast, it's really tricky. Even my husband, who's awesome and wonderful and supportive, he'd be devastated if I actually said to him, 'I'm planning on never drinking again.'

All of my problems are caused by drinking, but thinking of a life with no alcohol in it scares the shit out of me. Not only would I lose alcohol, but I feel like I would lose friends, I'd have to put up with shit from my family, and my relationship with my husband would change. So, if I want to keep all the relationships I have, I have to keep drinking.

I've only talked to my mum about the sexual abuse once since my childhood. We were drinking at the time, and she started saying that I turned into a naughty school girl before it started, and that's why the guy had his chance—basically implying I almost encouraged it. I love her to death, but I was so angry I was shaking. I lifted up my wine glass and actually felt like I might bloody hit her with it, I was that angry. I'll never speak with her about it again because I think I might lose my relationship with her if I do. I just have to live with the fact that she is naïve to it. Maybe it's too hard for her to look at. I don't know.

Sometimes I wonder how things would be different if the abuse never happened, because I think that really did change my path completely. I probably wouldn't have got into drinking as heavily. But I can't even imagine what it would have been like not drinking, given everything that had happened.

Part Five

MOVING ON

33.

The ultimate rebellion

One of the things I loved most about alcohol when I started drinking it in my teens, aside from the physical warmth and emotional numbness it gave me, was that it made me feel really cool. Drinking beer on the riverbank with my friends made me feel really cool. Buying cheap, sickly-sweet bubbly wine from the back entrance of the liquor store made me feel really cool. Getting plastered on my parents' gin made me feel really cool. Even vomiting my guts out every time I overdid it didn't *stop* me from feeling cool. Everything about alcohol made me feel cool. Cool and naughty and rebellious, and there was no better feeling as far as teenage me was concerned.

Teenage me loved nothing more than to be a little rebel. Railing against any sort of authority at home or school and desperately trying to assert myself as an independent person was my raison d'être. At a time in life when I still needed guidance and boundaries, I did not want to be told what to do or when to do it. Just ask my poor parents! I put them through the ringer in my teenage years by pushing back against almost every boundary that was imposed on me. I bunked off school, failed exams, lied about where I was going, snuck out of my bedroom window in the middle of the night, did a whole bunch of other naughty things that I'm not going to list here because they're too shameful, and drank. I drank and I drank and I drank.

Alcohol was the perfect accompaniment to my naughty, rebellious lifestyle. It was forbidden and alluring. It even tasted naughty, or so I thought. (Really it just tasted gross, but I translated gross to naughty in good rebellious fashion.) Overall I saw drinking alcohol as the perfect way for me to be everything that I wanted to be—strong, independent, feisty and cool. I'm still trying to be all of that now that I'm in my forties, but I've found a much better way to achieve it: ironically, it's by doing the very opposite of what I used to do—saying an enthusiastic 'no thanks' to alcohol, where I used to scream 'hell yes'.

Choosing not to pour alcohol down your throat on a regular basis in this alcohol-centric culture of ours is an utterly radical act. When alcohol is normalised and glorified at every turn and your entire environment almost demands that you drink, taking a stand and deciding *not* to imbibe is a hugely subversive and deeply rebellious thing to do. By choosing not to touch any alcohol, ever, I'm finally achieving what I've always wanted, except this time it's for real. That's because not drinking is the epitome of strong, independent, feisty and cool.

Drinking alcohol didn't make me strong; it diminished

my strength. Every night that I was under the influence I wasn't fully standing in my power with a clear head and feet planted firmly on the ground. Far from it. I was numbed to my emotions, vulnerable, distracted and disconnected from myself and the people around me.

Drinking alcohol didn't make me independent; it made me depend on something outside of myself. It made me rely on a liquid drug to feel confident and interesting, rather than being self-reliant and grounded in my natural state of being.

Drinking alcohol didn't make me feisty. With alcohol being so normalised, glorified, cheap and readily available, choosing to chuck it down my throat regularly just made me a sheep, blindly following the flock. I never stopped to properly question or examine what I was doing and whether it was truly serving me.

And drinking alcohol certainly didn't make me cool; it just made me blurry, sloppy, loud, slurry, clumsy, smelly, flippant, dismissive and (I'm pretty convinced of this now) boring. None of this equals cool.

Not drinking is the ultimate rebellion. Not drinking is so countercultural that the naughty teenager inside me is having a field day. I cannot believe how strong, independent and feisty I now feel (not to mention well rested and healthy). Every time I front up to an event and ask for a 'fizzy water, please', every time I say to the waiter 'the house-made soda, please', every time I'm at my local pub ordering a 'chamomile tea, please' (yes, I do that) and every time I'm searching around at a wedding for something non-alcoholic that isn't orange juice (gah), my inner rebel is punching the air, screaming, 'You go, girl!' It's delightful.

It's taken a bit of grit and determination to get to this

delightful place, of course. Transitioning away from being a boozer takes time and effort and it sure isn't a walk in the park. It's emotionally and physically draining and there are numerous stumbling blocks along the way. All the more reason why those of us who make it through the transition process to settle in and become contented non-drinkers truly are the epitome of feisty, strong and brave.

We're even feistier, stronger and braver when you consider that alcohol is the only drug that you might get judged harshly for *not* taking. Ever thought about that? Not only is our environment stacked massively in favour of drinking, but also it's stacked massively against *not* drinking. Say no to a drink and you're met with bemusement, disappointment or defensiveness. At best eyebrows get raised; at worst pressure gets applied. Questions like 'Why aren't you drinking?' get thrown around, as do statements like 'Just have one.' We find ourselves having to trot out excuses like 'I'm training for a marathon' or 'I'm on medication.' If we're really brave we'll tell the truth and say something like 'I've drunk my lifetime limit already' or 'I can't stop at one, so I'd rather not drink.' I prefer the honest approach, as it tends to shut the conversation down pretty quickly. And, as one of my Sober Stories interviewees at livingsober.org.nz, Luke, once said, 'It's way more interesting at dinner parties to say, "I'm a recovering crazy drunk and addict" than "No thanks, I'm driving."'

But why do we even need to explain or justify our actions? Why is it anyone's business what we choose to put in our glass? Would the same happen if we were saying no to a line of cocaine or a syringe full of heroin? Or any other drug you can name? It's crazy.

Non-drinkers can be judged, and not in a good way. We can be judged as being boring. We can be judged as being lame. We can be judged as having nasty skeletons in our closets. We can even be judged as being judgemental. And, when we're not being judged or accused, we're being pitied. Pitied for 'missing out', for not being able to have as much 'fun' as the drinkers. Well, I've got a few things to say about all of that.

First, non-drinkers aren't boring. As I said earlier, I think I was extremely boring back when I was necking wine daily. Boring is being half-present, repeating yourself, rattling on about stuff that isn't funny and having your attention span hijacked so you can't hold down a decent conversation.

Second, non-drinkers aren't lame. As I said earlier, I was lame when I was doing what everyone else was, despite it doing me no favours. Lame was allowing myself to be manipulated into constantly chucking a grade-one carcinogen down my throat.

Third, the skeletons in non-drinkers' closets aren't nasty; they're rich and intriguing. My skeletons give me depth, meaning, empathy and understanding. I love my skeletons because they got me to where I am today, which is a mighty fine place to be. And, anyway, who *doesn't* have skeletons in their closet?

Fourth, non-drinkers aren't judging drinkers. How could we possibly? We know what it's like to love booze. We also know that you can't judge the true nature of another person's drinking habit unless you're living with them 24/7. No, we're not judging. Most of the time we're just thinking to ourselves how gobsmackingly grateful we are that we don't drink anymore.

Which brings me to my final retort. Don't pity us. We don't need your compassion. We're good. But thanks anyway.

I honestly look at alcohol now as a cancer-causing poison, diluted with sugar and other flavourings to make it palatable, wrapped in fancy packaging with a price tag slapped on it. I don't hanker for it. I don't wish I could drink it. I don't envy people who do. The way I experience life now is so far removed from how I used to that I might as well be on another planet.

When I was boozing, it was like I was stuck at the back of a rock concert being pushed around by a squishy, smelly crowd, not able to see or hear the music properly. Now that I'm not drinking it's like I'm standing in the front row, right in front of the speakers with every drum beat and guitar lick pounding in my chest. Joyously stimulated, vibrantly alert, fantastically grounded and very much alive. 'Sobriety is full throttle,' writes Sarah Hepola in *Blackout: Remembering the things I drank to forget*.[1] 'No earplugs. No safe distance. Everything at its highest volume. All the complications of the world, vibrating your sternum.'

I've said it before and I'll say it again (and again, and again, until the cows come home), being a non-drinker is a mighty fine thing to be. But it did take some work to get here, and I'll go over what that can look like next.

34.

Clara

'I feel like my life has started again.'

My parents weren't heavy drinkers. They liked to have dinner parties and we'd go around to lots of people's houses, but I didn't see them get drunk much. They split up when I was at high school, Mum remarried and I then became the teenager from hell, probably wanting her attention. I probably made their lives a bit of a misery and I was given the option to board during the week at my school. It turned out for the better, but there was a lot of conflict in my teenage years.

Partying was very big at my boarding school. My first drink would have been when I was about thirteen. We all went to a tennis tournament and there was alcohol there, and it was incredibly naughty and fun. A couple of the boys got so drunk they vomited, and that was just unbelievably cool in our view. From then on most weekends were spent going to 'gatherings' or woolshed parties, sneaking alcohol into sleepovers. When I was fifteen, sixteen, Mum would let me take two beers or even a six-pack if I was lucky, and we'd ask older siblings if they could go and buy alcohol for us. We'd get a hip flask of Southern Comfort and some L&P, then pour half the L&P out and the Southern Comfort in. I think the smell of it now would make me retch.

I wasn't a heavy drinker then. I liked it and it was fun and silly, but I wasn't drinking that much and didn't get hangovers that badly. I had friends who would always go too far and vomit, but I mostly wasn't one of them.

I took a year out between high school and uni and went over to the north of England to work in a school. I went from being surrounded morning and night by my friends and family to being quite alone. I didn't recognise it at the time, but that was when I started getting quite bad anxiety. When the gap year finished I was so desperate to be back in a group of my friends that I chucked in my original plans to do teaching at Massey and enrolled to do law at Otago, which seemed like the most social uni and where most of my friends had gone.

I got into a very strong, passionate relationship with someone. It wasn't a healthy relationship and my anxiety got worse. My self-esteem and self-confidence had really taken a hit during my gap year, so I needed constant reassurance and stability. I tended to drink to cover my anxiety.

In my second year, everything was a struggle and I was just miserable and irritable all the time. I went to a GP and they diagnosed depression, and that's when I went on antidepressants. There were no questions about alcohol or exercise that I recall, which I think would be standard now.

I ended up quitting university, which I'm really ashamed of. I decided to follow a passion instead and did a diploma in beauty therapy. This was a good decision—I did really well at it, I made great new friends and my relationship was healthier. We got engaged and were very happy. We moved over to Australia and lived there for a year or two. We were in a crowd of heavy partiers again, and every weekend was spent either clubbing or having epic Sunday sessions. But then we broke up a few months before we were meant to get married and that was heartbreaking. We'd been together eight years and I was very young, and he just cut all lines of contact and I moved back to New Zealand.

I was in my late twenties and had to start all over again, and that was terrifying for me. It was a really hard time. I had a lot of panic attacks and anxiety during this time, and I went to a clinical psychologist for some help. They taught me some wonderful techniques on how to manage anxiety, but I do wonder whether it would have been better if I'd just drunk less.

I was a heavy drinker but so was everybody else—my normal drinking was very much everyone else's normal drinking. My mother was the only person who was concerned, but I would brush her off, saying it was normal and, 'Everyone else drinks like this.' It was normal to start drinking at 5 p.m. on a Friday, get home at 4 a.m., sleep until 11 a.m. and then have a second wind and another big night out. It didn't affect me physically, or so I thought. Eventually I moved to a smaller town to try and settle down. I ended up meeting my future husband and we married a couple of years later.

When I was trying to get pregnant a lot of my mates were trying to get pregnant as well, and so we'd have conversations around, 'Well if I get pregnant here, I can drink at Christmas.' Or, 'If I have the baby in November I'm going to be good for drinking at Christmas.' Then, when you discover you're pregnant, 'Christmas is going to be so boring this year.' I was very much of the mind that I was going to have a couple of drinks while I was pregnant, which I'm not proud of. I'd done all the research and was sure it was absolutely fine to have one or two. So I would have a glass of bubbles on Christmas Day and I would have perhaps a beer on a Friday night with my husband. Luckily I think your body tells you what you should and shouldn't be doing, and I never felt like having more than that, or needing more than that.

I was still on antidepressants, and when my kids were very young I was quite miserable. Being sleep-deprived was a really big trigger for my anxiety. My GP put me on a stronger drug, which works very well. I haven't had any panic attacks since taking it. I always wonder whether, if I'd been able to stop drinking for six months or so, my anxiety would have gone away without the need for this strong medication.

Overall my anxiety got worse after having children, and while now I look back and think the drinking was causing me anxiety, or was certainly a large part of it, at the time it seemed to be working to cut it out. Having a drink at 5 p.m. on the dot silenced the inner talk totally—one drink and it would just go, *Ahhhhh.* I'd be like, *Everything's gonna be fine. What was I worried about?* I'd be able to deal with things, do things with the kids or just relax at the end of the day.

I then got in the habit of sitting on the couch drinking wine by myself. If I felt that good after two glasses, why not have three? It was really dumb. I would sit up all hours drinking a whole bottle of wine, watching shit on the tele, then feeling hungover the next day. What was the point of that? That continued until I stopped drinking about three years later.

Towards the very end, I was starting to drink more than a bottle of wine in a night. Or I'd start with, like, two huge gins and then drink my bottle of wine. Our rule of not drinking Mondays and Tuesdays was starting to slide also, and I was white-knuckling those sober evenings. I didn't feel that drunk, but the next day I'd have a whopping hangover. Some mornings I could not get out of bed without being sick. Terrible nausea, terrible—just unable to eat or drink or do anything. A lot of people with a hangover can get out of bed, take a painkiller and drink a Powerade and just get on with it, whereas I could not move. If that's not a glaring red flag that my body was telling me to stop I don't know what is.

I knew that I had a drinking problem because there were days when I would google 'AA meetings' or 'how do you know you're an alcoholic?' All the quizzes that I did always put me into the heavy-drinking column. I was so confused as to why I would start the day saying I was never drinking again, but by 3 p.m. I'd be putting my wine in the fridge to chill. I would try to reason with myself. I'd think, *Well, everyone else drinks like me*. But, while the partying I did was just like everyone else, I was pretty secretive when it came to the drinking far too much while sitting on the couch. None of my friends knew about that. I vividly remember texting to one of my mum friends, 'Why is parenting so much easier when you've had a wine?' and she wrote back, 'It just is.'

Eventually the shit hit the fan; the hangovers got out of control and everything revolved around drinking. I ended up having a huge night out at a party and behaving like a complete idiot, which ended in a whopping fight with my husband. The next morning he asked me to choose between our family and drinking. It was an easy choice.

I didn't know how to stop, but I certainly knew that I couldn't do it on my own, because I had already tried to moderate. I'd tried to do a month off, and lasted only six days. I'd tried to do only weekends. It was really scary. I knew I had to be humble and ask for help. Fate played a hand and a wonderful friend told me her story, got things in motion and got me into AA.

There are hundreds of ways to quit, but for me AA worked. Oh my God, it's so awesome! It's just unbelievable. The whole point of AA is that you go every day for the first six weeks, or at least attempt to. And that was amazing, because each day I was able to share my story, listen to other people's stories and understand that, yeah, I really did have a problem. You're in these rooms with people who are a complete cross-section of society, and we all have one thing in common: we have an illness called alcoholism. It's humbling.

Drinking had been my favourite thing. The only way that I thought I could feel happy. The only way I could laugh and have fun. The only way. To me it was like saying goodbye to a best friend. I just couldn't understand how I was going to live my life without alcohol. I still feel like that two and a half years later. So that's why I still do that 'one day at a time' thing. If the thought of *Holy shit, I am never drinking alcohol again* gets too much, I just think, *No, no, no. It's just today. I'm just not drinking today.* It does get easier and these thoughts come less and less.

I wouldn't have stopped without the ultimatum. I needed to hit rock bottom before I made a change. I needed to know that I was not going to see my children every day if I didn't do this. And that was such an easy choice for me. I was very lucky—for some, getting sober can take years.

My life isn't any worse than what it was beforehand; in fact it is unbelievably better. I've got a job that I'm good at. My children have a mother who is fully present in their lives, not reading the ends of books quickly so she can get back to her wine. My head is so much clearer. Maybe I'll finish my degree. Maybe I'll get fluent in te reo. Maybe I'll write my own book. At the age of 40 I feel like my life has started again and I am so grateful this has happened to me.

35.

Anyone can

If I had a dollar for every time someone who has changed their relationship with alcohol said 'If I can do it, anyone can', I'd be a very rich woman. Those words are so frequently uttered by people who have stopped steadily drinking they've almost become meaningless. Which is a shame given it's such a powerful and compelling statement. Just seven short words, but used in this context they are drenched in meaning. They convey pride and power, but also a measure of incredulity, almost as if the person uttering them can't quite believe what they've done in turning their lives around. Why not? Because they genuinely thought they'd never be able to do it.

Most of us who have quit drinking *used* to think our booze habits were so deeply ingrained we'd never shift them. We couldn't imagine life without our 'best friend', alcohol. We were terrified at the thought of resisting cravings, socialising sober, celebrating events and dealing with emotions in the raw for the rest of our lives. Perhaps we also thought our mental-health issues were too difficult to manage, or our childhood trauma too awful to get over. Whatever the circumstances surrounding our drinking, most of us genuinely thought it would be impossible to change things, and that we'd never sort it out. Until, that is, we did.

We dug deep and worked like demons to shift our thinking, form new habits, develop new coping mechanisms, work on our underlying issues and fundamentally change. Through grit, sweat, blood and tears, we did it. Fighting and persevering until we got to a place where we felt happy and free. Where finally, when most of the hard work was done and the coast was clear, we looked back on where we came from and uttered the words, 'If I can do it, anyone can.' Incredulous, yes, but also proud. And most of all, hopeful. Hopeful for all the others still struggling. You can see that hope reflected in the final two words of the statement: 'anyone can'.

I truly believe this to be true. Anyone can shift their drinking habit. Absolutely anyone. Everyone has the ability to change. No matter what happened in your past or what's present in your current circumstances. No matter how terrifying your fears or deep-rooted your beliefs. You. Can. Change. Hundreds of thousands of people around the globe have done it. To join them, you just have to believe you can do it.

'Hope is everything,' says clinical psychologist Karen Nimmo. 'You've got to feel hopeful that you can move forward and life can be better before you can make a lasting change. If you're really up for doing things differently, you can do it. No one should rule themselves out of being able to make a change and improve their lives.'

Nimmo knows what she's talking about. She's been helping people turn their lives around for decades, and in that time has witnessed some incredible transformations. 'Change is possible really quickly if you're up for it. I think it's really important that we send that message because often, especially when people have to deal with big issues, we are sold the story that it will take years. No. If you're really up for making your life better, you can do it, and you can do it more quickly, probably, than people realise.'

Nimmo says that, alongside hope, having an open mindset is key, as is the need to take the action required to form new habits. 'It's not enough to talk about it, or to understand it. You've got to make the small changes required in order to get to where you want to go. If you have somewhere in mind that is not where you are now, the gap is yours to work on.'

Alcohol counsellor Crystal McLean has been helping women address their drinking issues for many years. She's also seen some incredibly powerful transformations in her time. 'I know this can work. I've seen absolute miracles. I'm saying this from my heart. I've seen absolute miracles of women turning their lives around, and bringing back their power. Because with alcohol we might feel powerful while we're in the midst of it. But it actually takes our power away.'

This is the problem, of course. One of the biggest things to go out the window when we're deep in a boozy hell-hole is any sense of hope, pride or self-belief. When I was at the end of my drinking days, stuck and miserable, having battled for years to try to control my drinking, my self-belief was utterly shot. Any sense of inner strength or resilience that I may have once had was diminished to next to nothing. I felt like a weak, pathetic failure. How could I not? Time and again I'd made deals with myself that I had broken. I'd promise myself that I'd only have one glass, but then I'd have five. I'd promise myself I'd take a month off, but would only last a week. I flip-flopped around in my head day after day. Making a promise, then breaking it. Vowing to change, then not. It was an awful place to be. Confusing and miserable. And the worst, most disempowering thing of all? I had no one to blame but myself. It was my hand opening the bottle. It was my arm lifting the glass. It was all me. How could I possibly ever find the hope to turn things around?

Eventually I found it on the morning after my last-ever binge. A little glimmer of hope came to me through floods of tears when (as I wrote in my introduction) I had that monumental thought, *The problem isn't me. The problem is the alcohol.* I seized on that glimmer of hope, used it to tap into the tiny amount of strength I had remaining, and made my decision to quit. It was utterly terrifying. Truly, deeply terrifying. But I held onto my little inner glimmer of hope, and boosted it with the vague notion I had that it was possible to become a happy non-drinker. This I'd gleaned from looking at the occasional famous person I knew had quit. As tragic as it sounds, I'd see former drinkers like Rob Lowe and Keith Urban on the red carpet on E! channel and notice they seemed really happy. I knew they'd both quit their nasty drinking habits, yet they seemed content, smiling like life without alcohol was okay. How they'd done it, I had no idea, but they showed me that it could be done. I thought, *If they can do it, I can too.*

That's the other thing to grasp onto if your personal hope and sense of self isn't quite there yet, and your inner strength is shot. Look around and find some lamplighters—people who have quit drinking and don't appear miserable. There are so many. Look for famous celebrities like I did if you must. Look for local television personalities or media stars. Look for people writing books (like this one!), sharing posts and photos on social media, and articles and blog posts on recovery websites. Look around in your real life—you may be lucky enough to have a role model in your extended family or community. Look for us and look hard *at* us. None of us are miserable about our non-drinking status. We're not bereft; we're just living. We've all done the hard work, we've all got to a comfortable place, and we all want nothing more but to shine a light and show others the way. Follow us on social media, get our books, listen to our podcasts, join our online communities. And constantly remind yourself, if we can do it, anyone can. Anyone.

36.

Alix

*'I consider myself worthy for
the first time in 52 years.'*

I had a very difficult upbringing. I never laid eyes on my
father; I only had a mother, and she suffered from a
significant mental illness that impaired her ability to be
a healthy and fully functioning parent. We had no family
around as she was new to New Zealand, and she had few
friends, so there was never any supportive or alternative
parental figure throughout my formative years. I did have
a brother, but when I was eight he was sent into permanent
care and I was left alone with this woman. Although I called
her Mother, I never felt like she was my mother. Equally, I
never felt like a child . . . anyone's child.

As such, there was nothing resembling any normal
form of parenting and I felt no connection to her or anyone
whatsoever. I have no animosity though, because I think

my mother's story was a very, very difficult one, and she did the best she could. As a child you don't question a lot because you only know what you know. But, looking back, it was incredibly sad. Children shouldn't grow up without love, children shouldn't grow up without nurturing, and every child needs at least one person they can rely on or be able to turn to.

Part of her mental illness was having episodes of rage, so at night time she would bang loudly on my bedroom door, screaming and trying to get into my bedroom. Incredibly frightened, I used to push my bed up against the door so she couldn't get in. Eventually I learned to climb out the window and hit the streets, so I actually became a street-wise kid very young. I used to sleep on bench seats hidden from view. That was where I felt safe.

When I was a pre-teen I got placed under the care of a family, which was my first experience of having mother- and father-type figures, and I was like a big sister to their young children. It was mind-blowing for me, and for the first time in my life I felt happy and that I belonged. I got away from the horrendous home life, I was taken off the streets, I was made to feel loved and included. But little did I know the father was actually a paedophile, and I was his target. He was respected in the community, and he deliberately chose me because I was clearly a vulnerable child. That sexual abuse went on for two years.

So, between the lack of nurturing through childhood and that horrific experience within the family, when I finally tasted alcohol for the first time, aged twenty, it went downhill very quickly from there. I realised that this wonderful new drink that I'd never experienced numbed things really, really well. It zoned me out.

I got into a circle of friends where drinking was the be all and end all. I was a bit of a wild child at that time, because I'd got away from the dysfunction of childhood and was free to live my life. Oh my God, it was like, *Hello, World! Wild Child has arrived. Watch out!* I was heavily involved in a sports club, and alcohol was a huge part of that environment—it was very enabling and encouraging. If you weren't drinking, people were like, 'Come on, come on, we're all drinking. Don't be a nana. Don't be a sad sack.' Not that any persuasion was really necessary. I was normally first at the bar, and I just drank and drank and drank.

I was very much the high-functioning alcoholic, from the point of view that I had responsible jobs and I did them really well. I didn't drink during the day. I didn't drink on the job. Even if there was a luncheon with alcohol I wouldn't partake. I was very much the five o'clock drinker, downing cheap cask wine or vodka, and in really large quantities. What I didn't realise for a long time was that what I was doing was ensuring that I went to bed basically comatose. I couldn't bear for my head to hit the pillow conscious. Because all the sick things that had happened in my childhood had happened at night when I was in bed. And that went on for 25 years. I can barely remember a night in those 25 years that I was 'aware' when my head hit the pillow. It was how I survived the memories—by blocking them.

I was married twice. The first man I married was a good man and we genuinely did love each other. He was quite a drinker himself and that kind of made it too easy, too acceptable. We weren't going to question each other's habits, because most other aspects of our life together were going okay. Then we decided to have a child and I desperately, desperately wanted to be a mother. I think in my mind I felt that motherhood would cure all the sins of the past. And I also believed it would be the catalyst for me to stop drinking, and that it would be really easy for me to do that because I would have what I always wanted. To be able to give and receive love unconditionally. But I had four miscarriages in the space of two years. Each miscarriage was beyond devastating, not only for the normal reasons that it's devastating, but also because it brought back that sense of loss and abandonment. So after each miscarriage I went straight back to alcohol, drinking even harder to compensate and numb myself even further. In my head that was the answer; that was going to cure the pain.

That relationship finally broke down because we didn't talk about our losses, we didn't face it. The spiral of grief just increased to a point where we split up. It was an intensely sad time.

Then I was incredibly blessed to find the second man I married. The love of my life, the man of my dreams and my whole world. We were so in love, a match made in heaven, and I felt like the luckiest woman on earth. And it mitigated to a degree the losses of my babies. He wasn't a big drinker at all. He was very well known and respected in the community, so after we got together I made my drinking far more private. I felt I couldn't be seen with this highly respected man, getting sloshed at functions and events. I would top up before we went out, so it looked like when we were out I was only having one or two. And if I looked like I was a bit shonky on it people would think I was a lightweight instead of knowing I'd skulled a glass or three of vodka before I left home. And when I got home I'd top up with another two or three. My husband knew how I was drinking, but his love was so deep, and he understood the reasons why I did it, so it was never discussed.

Then two years into our marriage we were told that he had an incurable form of cancer—one of the deadliest cancers there is. It should have been a wake-up call to kick the drink, because life was about to get so much more difficult than either of us had ever imagined. But the grip of the addiction was so huge by then that I didn't have the strength to fight it.

Within days he started chemotherapy, and within a few months he went through a stem-cell transplant. The transplant meant a month-long stay for him in a hospital out of town, with me staying in a motel opposite. I was with him from seven o'clock in the morning until nine o'clock at night as he went through absolute hell. Each night I went back to the motel and drank myself senseless, crying on the bathroom floor. The bottle was my only comfort. I didn't know how else to get through the pain of seeing what my husband was going through, and knowing I was going to lose him. It's crazy because it was the worst thing in the world I could do to myself, but it was the only thing I knew. I was an addict, but at that stage no horrific experience could bring me to my knees to change.

We were very lucky that he lived for seven more years, but they were seven incredibly difficult years with his health.

A year before he died he started to go downhill rapidly, and I started drinking more—over half a bottle of vodka a night, barely diluted. I had so much self-loathing. I would promise myself that I wouldn't do it again, that I'd stop, that today was going to be a different day, but it never was. I was absolutely lost to it. And moderation was impossible.

Then one night, 1 January 2014, I had another massive binge session. I got up like any other morning, hungover as hell, feeling like shit, with no idea if I'd had dinner or what I'd said or done the night before. My dear husband ever so gently said to me, 'How are you feeling?' He didn't normally ask how I was feeling, because I got really good at hiding it and pretending I was fine. So I said, 'Oh, I'm fine! I'm fine,' and he said to me, 'Honey, I'm really, really worried about you.' I asked, 'Why?' And he said, 'The amount you're drinking really worries me. You're drinking more than you've ever drunk, faster than you've ever drunk it.' And I was like, *Oh holy shit, I've never been confronted before.* And then he said to me, 'If you keep this up you're going to kill yourself.' And you know, that statement didn't work for me because I didn't care. I didn't love myself—I never had. I had spent 47 years feeling unworthy and unlovable, so that wasn't the kicker. And I think he sensed that pretty quickly because there wasn't any shock value. So then he said the thing that finally got to me: 'If I had come down with an infection in the middle of the night you wouldn't have been able to take me to hospital. I could have died.'

Woah! That slapped me in the face like a massive avalanche had hit me. Because I suddenly knew that the man I loved more than life itself, including more than I loved myself, was having his life put at risk, and his life was already delicately hanging by a thread. That was the profound turning point, and I knew in my heart of hearts I had to do something immediately. I couldn't allow another night being written off, him potentially needing to be rushed to hospital, and me not being able to do that. So that was it. I have never touched a drop of alcohol since that day.

It was hard work with yearnings and cravings, but much worse was the news we received at that time. Four months after I quit we were told that my husband had weeks—months at best—to live. But I didn't drink. For the next five months I watched my husband dying. Didn't drink. I watched him die in my arms. Didn't drink. I spoke at his funeral. Didn't drink. And how I managed that was by honouring my husband. In my determination to keep honouring that wonderful man, I thought to myself, *If he was able to love me through all that drinking, all that drunkenness, I can keep honouring him by continuing not to drink.*

It was seven months after he died, and seven months of running on adrenaline, that I finally hit the wall. I was literally brought to my knees, and the temptation of alcohol was probably at its greatest, but such was my determination that I didn't drink. However, I did recognise I needed some help. This is a journey that nobody should travel alone. And that's when a therapist was found and I started really working on myself. My therapist told me, 'Over 70 per cent of people who are sexually abused become addicted to alcohol.' She pretty much saved my life, but I had to do the work and I had to be prepared to look at demons.

It was really gritty, hard work. Facing why I started

drinking, facing up to yucky, yucky hard stuff that I had spent my drinking life burying, numbing myself from. But after doing it my life completely and utterly transformed.

I consider myself worthy for the first time in 52 years. I don't blame myself now for picking up the bottle, but that took a long time to understand because both childhood trauma and alcohol distort your mind, so it takes a long time to actually come to grips with the reality. Many years in fact. And the reality is: my childhood was not my fault. The sexual abuse was not my fault. Addiction was not my fault. Alcohol was a tool that I found and thought to be successful at that time. And it is successful at numbing, if numbing is what you want. But numbing is not what anybody needs. You might think you do, but it's not what anyone needs—not ever.

I used to think of drinking as self-care when times were tough. Drink wine, eat chocolate, watch chick flicks—it all seemed to go hand in hand. Or eat comfort food, drink comfortable old alcohol—yet it's all just escapism. We can't spend our whole lives escaping from reality. We're not being authentic, and we're not facing up to what is actually an incredible life and an incredible world out there.

At the end of the day, there is no amount of shit, no amount of obstacles, no amount of reasons that are enough to keep drinking when it's spiralling out of control. We are all worthy of so much better. I have conquered shit, and dealt with obstacles, and yes it was fucking hard, and still is at times, but that is reality. But, if I can do it, anyone can do it, and trust me it is absolutely worth it.

37.

Recovery 101

Now I'm going to do something crazy, which is to summarise the recovery process in around 4000 words. It's a bit of a ridiculous thing to do given that changing drinking habits is an incredibly complicated and multifaceted process that plays out differently for everyone. However, among all the various unique and personal aspects that make up each individual's journey, there are many similar issues and common scenarios that arise. We all have to deal with cravings. We all have to learn how to socialise sober. We all have to shift our hardwired thinking. We all have to learn how to sit with uncomfortable emotions. And we all have to formulate new habits.

I'm fairly well versed in each of these recovery processes, having not only gone through it all myself, but also having borne intimate witness to loads of others going through it as well—most notably in my role as the community manager at livingsober.org.nz, where thousands of members have been posting daily for many years about what they're going through. So, bearing in mind that I am summarising and generalising massively, here is a breakdown of some of the main things you will encounter when transitioning from being a drinker to being a non-drinker (if that's what you want to do).

Cravings

They will come and they will suck. Cravings manifest in the physical body, but they also feature very loudly in the mind. So while your body will yearn and pine for its chemical fix, making you feel itchy and uncomfortable, your brain will also throw the biggest bloody wobbly you have heard for a very long time. My cravings mostly consisted of a wall of words inside my head trying to convince me to drink. Just a constant stream of thoughts coming at me—in my own voice, no less—urging me to pick up a drink. Justifications, excuses, reasons, ploys. Sometimes it would go on for hours. Nobody else could hear it, and they couldn't tell by looking at my face that it was going on. It was like an excruciating private torture chamber inside my mind. Not fun at all.

The good news is that there is a way to silence cravings forever. The not-so-good news is that it takes a while. But it does work and, if you stick at it, it's a permanent fix. The solution? Ignore them. If you ignore the cravings, hard as it is at first, they will slowly fade and lessen over time to where they hardly pop up at all. I'm over eight years sober now and I can't remember the last time a thought entered my brain trying to convince me to drink. Certainly it was well over five years ago. I'm reluctant to put an exact timeframe on when cravings end as it's likely to be different for everyone (as are most things in recovery, and in life), but I can guarantee you that, if you resist and ignore them for long enough, eventually the cravings will stop. That's the long-term fix: resist and they'll fade to nothing. But what to do in the short term while you're resisting and being tortured in your own mind?

Firstly, think of HALTS. If you're having a craving ask yourself whether you are Hungry, Angry, Lonely, Tired or Stressed? Often it's one of these sensations or emotions that is causing us to crave. What can you do to address your need that isn't imbibing alcohol? Maybe you need to eat, let off steam, reach out to connect with someone, have a nap or a bubble bath, or do something lovely and nurturing.

Next, think: *Delay and distract.* Get busy to get your mind off the craving. I used to clean the house hard-out. Other people go for a run (good for the thighs!), or do some other exercise or mind-occupying task. Do whatever you need to in order to take your mind off the urge. Cravings tend to come in waves, so if you delay and distract for long enough the intensity will pass and you can relax a little. Sometimes the best thing is to go to bed. Really early if you have to. Like, reeeeeeaaaalllllyy early.

It's also helpful to talk about your craving out loud. Say, 'I'm having an intense craving right now' to whoever is in the room with you, or simply out loud to yourself. Watch and see if that helps take some of the heat out of your inner voice. I can vividly remember saying out loud just a few days after I quit, 'There's a voice in my head trying to convince me to drink.' It really helped me to feel less stressed about my awful inner dialogue.

Finally, visualise. Push your thoughts forward through the evening and visualise yourself climbing into bed sober.

Visualise yourself laying your clear head on the pillow and sleeping well all night. Visualise yourself waking up hangover-free in the morning, feeling so good and so proud of yourself for not having crumbled and taken a drink the night before. Nobody ever woke up regretting *not* having a drink the night before. Visualisation is a really powerful tool to get you to that lovely, satisfied moment.

One final note about cravings. If you stop drinking and find yourself shaking uncontrollably, sweating profusely, vomiting endlessly or seeing things that aren't there—please get yourself to a doctor quick smart. Alcohol is one of the most dangerous drugs to detox from, so be ready to call for professional help if needed.

Socialising sober

Going out and mixing with others without liquid courage can be hard work at first. I felt like a total weirdo going to social events right after I quit, like I had a big neon sign flashing above my head that said 'Not Drinking!!' and everyone was looking at me sideways. I was silly to feel so self-conscious, given what I now know, which is that most people don't care if you're drinking or not. (Some do, but it's best not to focus too much on them.) Having said that, it makes perfect sense that we feel so deeply out of sorts when we start entering situations that have for most of our lives been accompanied by alcohol. It's no small deal to be going out and getting amongst it with only soda water for company, especially when everyone else around is glugging their ethanol, so first and foremost remind yourself every minute you can that you're freaking brave and amazing for even doing it.

One thing I found really useful early on when heading into social situations was to make a mental list of all the things that were fun or worthwhile about the event ahead. Things that weren't about what liquid I had in my glass. I would formulate a list in my mind of things to focus on. *This party is about celebrating Simon's promotion, the end of the working year and the kids having a Secret Santa. This barbecue is about summer arriving, my new dress and catching up with neighbours. This dinner is about checking out a hot new restaurant, showing off my new hairdo and seeing old friends. This wedding is about a young couple's love, the yummy food and dancing to cheesy music.* There are always things to be found that make an event worthwhile or special, and if you focus on those it can help take some of the heat out of the fact you feel weird for not drinking. If you can't find one single good thing to focus on, then that's usually a sign that you should be staying at home (and there's absolutely no shame in that).

If, however, you have got reason to head out, go prepared. Take your own non-alcoholic drink if it's a BYO event, or be ready with what you're going to order from the bar or waiter. Be bold and take ownership of your alcohol-free drink. Ditch the straw that they so often seem to hand out with non-alcoholic drinks (we're not kids, FFS) and be specific. If you want fresh limes, ask for them. If you want no ice, say so. If you want to use a wine glass, use it. Stemware is not solely reserved for liquids with percentage points.

And finally, have an exit plan. When you feel it's time to go, don't hesitate—go. If you're driving other people to the venue, warn them that you might slip out early and they should be prepared to make their own way home. Tell your significant other that you may go quietly at some point, and not to worry, you'll see them at home. Again, there is no shame in leaving a party early and heading home to snuggle the cat and have a nice mug of tea while catching up on some late-night tele, knowing you're going to get a great night's sleep and wake up blissfully hangover-free. That never gets old.

Brain retraining

This one is crucial, and we all have to work hard at doing it because we've got so many beliefs hardwired into us about the supposed benefits of alcohol. Thoughts we've been thinking for so many years they've worn deep grooves in our grey matter. The ones telling us that alcohol is the 'treat' or 'reward' that we 'deserve' for working hard. That alcohol is the best way to relax, have fun, host, celebrate, commiserate or grieve. So many lies that we've been constantly told by marketers and have repeated so often to ourselves and each other that they seem impossible to shift. They're not impossible to shift at all. You just have to do it in a very concerted way.

Every time a hardwired belief or positive thought about alcohol pops into your head, stop yourself, identify the thought (see it clearly for what it is), challenge it, remind yourself of the truth and then reframe it. For example, if you find yourself thinking, *How will I possibly enjoy this party if I'm not drinking?* Stop! Identify the thought and see it for what it is: *I'm just feeling insecure and that's an old idea about what constitutes enjoyment.* Then challenge it: *That's bullshit.* (Always the best challenge to any hardwired belief about alcohol. Brief and to the point.) Remind yourself of the truth: *The last party I went to I got so drunk I made a total dick of myself, which wasn't fun at all.* Then reframe it: *I'm going to enjoy this party because I've got new shoes on, my sister's out for the first time since she had her baby and Dan's bringing his guitar.* Stop, identify, challenge, remind, reframe. That's not a fancy acronym (SICRR?) but it works as a brain-retraining process. I'll put it a little more simply just to ram it home. Thoughts aren't facts. Challenge what you're thinking about alcohol and actively work to turn your thoughts around. Get help by reading blogs and books on this very topic. Jason Vale's *Kick the Drink . . . Easily!* and Allen Carr's *The Easy Way to Stop Drinking* were two books that really worked for me. Anything by Annie Grace is also very powerful.

Brain retraining takes hard work, determination, time and practice, practice, practice. Sometimes you just have to fake it until you make it. But never stop believing that you will turn your thinking around. You will. Because the truth always wins out in the end.

Sitting with uncomfortable emotions

There's no getting away from this one. Alcohol numbs emotions, so taking it away (or reducing it greatly) means you will have to feel them in all their raw glory. And, boy, can that hurt. Sadness and anger—they suck. Frustration and disappointment—they're not fun. I spent my entire drinking career (twenty-plus years) avoiding having to feel any such things, not that I knew this was what I was doing at the time. I thought I was just a party girl who liked to have fun. I didn't realise I was an A-grade emotion-avoider until I got sober and got so goddam emotional. Crikey, I was all over the show for quite a few months, lurching from one emotional state to the other. It was like I was strapped into a crazy rollercoaster ride called 'human experience' that I couldn't get off. Thankfully things eventually calmed down. I got used to riding the waves of emotion and managing the mood fluctuations that come naturally in life. I learned that sadness and anger (and all those other supposedly 'negative' feelings) don't kill you, they're generally there for a reason, and allowing yourself to fully feel them makes them easier to deal with. Sounds so cheesy, doesn't it? But it really is true.

Going through a hard or gritty time without reaching for a million bottles of wine (as I would have in the past) not only makes it quicker to process things, but also makes things clearer and easier to understand when looking back in hindsight. If I think back now to some of the hard times I've encountered since I stopped drinking, the tears I shed or stress or discomfort I experienced at the time makes perfect sense. It feels right. My reactions were appropriate—they fitted the severity of what I was going through at the time and accurately reflected how significant those events were. Even if at the time it was uncomfortable and I might have wanted to avoid or escape the difficulties (with my former best friend, vino), by simply allowing myself to sit with my feelings and experience them fully I felt more in touch with what was going on and, as a result, more resolved about what was happening. As time goes on, everything starts to appear more manageable, and it leads to a lovely overall feeling of calm as the years roll on.

What I've learned since I've been working on becoming a fully emotional human being (rather than one who constantly numbs and avoids emotions) is this: it's best not to panic when the shit hits the fan and you start to feel uncomfortable emotionally. Don't automatically reach for something to make the pain go away. Slow down and trust that the feelings are there for a reason. Try to adopt an open mindset and be curious about what your emotions are telling you. Understand the importance of letting yourself fully experience what you're going through. Trust that time will help and you'll look back and be grateful that you allowed yourself to get through with a clear head. Be gentle and kind to yourself. Self-care is really important.

And if things are too monumental to get through alone, reach out and get some professional help. There are loads of lovely trained people dotted all around our communities, just waiting to put their skills to use and help. Shit happens to all of us, all the time. There's no avoiding it. So don't try. Get stuck in and deal with it. It hurts at the time, but it is far, far better in the long run. Future you will thank you. Trust me on that.

Developing new habits

This step in the recovery process is really important and it starts from day one and never ends. Life shifts and changes when alcohol is out of the picture. All that time and energy you used to spend thinking about alcohol, planning to drink, obtaining alcohol, drinking alcohol and recovering from alcohol is freed up. Depending on your intake levels this can result in a LOT of free time and energy. And money! That's the great news. You'll have more coin in your pocket to spend on treats and things. So get thinking and get ready for some new habits and self-care practices to enter your life. We need lots of them, and they change over time, so be prepared to be adaptable. These can be little changes at first, and perhaps big ones over time. And what might work in the first month to nourish, occupy and ground you might not be so effective in the fifth year. It's a constant and ever-evolving process; there's no getting away from it and it can be hard work at times. Thankfully, it's also rewarding.

Don't be shy about treating yourself. Think of what you'd like to spend some of that former booze money on. Fancy replacement drinks, for starters. Glossy magazines perhaps? Fresh flowers or new guitar strings? Te reo lessons or surf-lifesaving classes? It's not so much about the material things you are buying; it's more that every purchase sends a little message to yourself that you are worth treating. Each transaction is a reminder that you're brave and amazing for reshaping your life and deserve some recognition.

Develop new relaxation triggers. My personal favourite is putting on comfy pants. The kind of pants that you'd never wear outside of the house but they're so super comfy you can't bear parting with them. I tend to do this regularly at 5 p.m. Other relaxation triggers that work for me are turning my phone to silent, lighting a scented candle or playing a favourite album while doing some cooking. Your relaxation trigger may be spending some time in the garden, having a bubble bath or watching *The Chase* with a delicious mug of creamy coffee. These are genuinely relaxing actions, not the false sense of ease that comes with drinking alcohol.

Get busy making plans to fill time. Maybe going to movies on your own is the ultimate treat. It is mine, especially at random times of the week like 11 a.m. on a Tuesday. There's nothing more indulgent and relaxing, and I never feel guilty about it or weird for doing it on my own. Walk on the beach, crochet a shawl, read all those novels you've never had time to read, get into crossfit or country music or complicated board games. If you're a social creature, join a sewing club, go trampolining with your kids or form a coffee group with friends. Push yourself out there, even if you're feeling a bit vulnerable and raw. It'll pay off in the long run. I could list a million things here, but you get the picture. Think back to your childhood—what did you enjoy as a kid? Maybe that's something to get back into.

Make sure there's some kind of body movement in your week—even if it's just walking the dog regularly or lumbering through a YouTube yoga lesson on your living-room floor. Move, stretch, bounce, lean, sweat. One foot in front of the other. Stuff. Just do stuff.

And think about your spiritual life and how that might be boosted. This could be church or faith, mindfulness or meditation, nature or music—whatever spirituality means to you. It can be a tricky thing to consider, but it's worthwhile paying some attention to as it's a crucial aspect of wellness, I think.

While we're talking about life shifting and changing, it's

also worth noting that you may find that some relationships are altered after you decide to re-examine your drinking. Whether this is romantic relationships or friendships, it can be hard coming to terms with this movement in your life. These relationship changes will only happen if they really need to, and you'll likely be aware, deep down, of this fact. Go gently, keep reminding yourself why you're making such a big life change and trust that over time lovely new relationships based on common values and goals will fall into place. Which leads me to my final point.

Communicating with people who get it

This is so important. It's vital to find people who understand exactly what you're going through because they've either already been through it or are currently going through it as well. We need people who understand. People who are wired the same. People who can relate to feeling uncomfortable about alcohol and looking at making changes. People who get that it's not as simple as saying, 'Just have one drink if you're that worried.' (Something my husband, bless him, used to say to me.)

Not everyone struggles with booze; there are those who enjoy a very casual relationship with the stuff and don't spend any time worrying or feeling guilty about it. In this context, they're not your people. My husband is an amazing, lovely, fully supportive and incredibly kind guy, but he could never really understand the battle I had going on in my head and the depth of the transformation I was going through. Thankfully, I found a community of like-minded people through my blog, and was able to converse with them daily for the first few years. We shared, empathised, commiserated, advised, suggested, celebrated and championed each other non-stop as we lurched through. This is what you need. Find your recovery people. Find them in support groups in your community. Find them in your wider family or work environment. Find them in private Facebook groups or anonymous online communities like livingsober.org.nz and others that exist around the internet. Find them anywhere; I don't care where, just find them. You need them and they need you. We all need each other. Because although our stories regarding alcohol are different, by sharing our individual truths, together we are stronger.

38.

Louise

*'Alcohol was there for me for sad,
mad, bad and glad—for everything.'*

I grew up in Australia in the 1970s, and both my parents
were heavy drinkers. Dad was definitely an alcoholic, and I
would call my mother an alcoholic too, actually, or at least a
problem drinker. They drank heavily every night and fought
constantly. My younger brother and sister and I lived in fear.
I knew it wasn't normal, and it wasn't good, because the
heavy drinking went hand in hand with domestic violence
and abuse. The beatings I got from my dad were vicious and
prolonged. Ironically, he didn't hit us much if he was
drinking—it was mainly when he was sober. Mum was the
opposite—she was nasty when she was drinking and quite
pleasant when sober. We all knew not to talk to her after
6 p.m. as by then she was sloshed, bitchy and really negative.
She was prone to a bit of violence when she drank, too.

I started drinking with Mum and Dad pretty early, probably when I was about eleven. Around the dinner table, have a glass of wine with the roast dinner sort of thing. It might have been watered down, but I do remember getting pissed with them. I started sneaking drinks at about twelve, when they went out. I remember one day sitting on the front step, and they'd gone out and I'd had a very stressful day—I was only twelve, but I was stressed out. And I remember thinking, *Oh thank God they've gone so I can have a beer and a cigarette*, sitting on the front step like an old woman.

I left home at fifteen and that's when I started drinking every chance I could get my hands on it. Binge drinking on a Friday or Saturday night, whatever I could afford. I would drink quite heavily until I blacked out. I did slowly learn how to . . . I wouldn't say moderate, but rather than vomiting and blacking out all the time I learned how to tolerate alcohol a bit better.

I went to rehab at nineteen because I'd made a total mess of my life. My mother had also gone into rehab, and it was very obvious to everyone that my father was a screaming, raging alcoholic. So you know, the game was up and I was very aware that alcohol was a major problem in my life and in my family's life. So I put myself in rehab, which was a very good thing for me to do. It planted all the seeds of recovery.

I stayed sober for eleven months, but then I went back to drinking, with the full knowledge that I was an alcoholic and I knew how to get sober. I was quite cocky about it actually. I was just like, *Well, I'll give up when I have to. And in the meantime I'll just kind of carry on until I can't get away with it anymore.*

I don't know how I managed to do anything, I got myself into so much trouble. I did actually manage to get an education and a career and all that sort of stuff. It was pretty haphazard, but I lurched along in a half-hearted manner through my twenties. I think when you're young your body can cope with a lot more. And in a lot of ways I really needed alcohol. It was my medicine for everything. It was my crutch for life, because I was pretty messed up from my family environment. I needed it to medicate myself, to calm myself down. It served a great purpose, really, in lots of ways. Alcohol was there for me for sad, mad, bad and glad—for everything.

When I was working, I'd go to the pub with colleagues as soon as we'd finished for the day, and stay there as late as anyone would stay with me. I wasn't interested in drinking with people who were just going to have one or two, I wanted my friends to be massive session drinkers. I looked at people in terms of *Would they drink with me or wouldn't they?* I was so black and white about it. My relationships with men were formed around how much they drank. I preferred it if they drank slightly more than me, because then I wouldn't look too bad. It all changed when I became a mum, because it became about my routine with the child. That was in my thirties, when I was constantly trying to give up and not doing very well most of the time.

I met Mike when I was doing yet another sober stint. He was different and special, but I was weak and wobbly in my sobriety and soon went back to drinking cheap rosé like a fish. He was confounded at how utterly pissed I would get in a short amount of time because I always hid exactly how much I was drinking through a complicated system of only pouring from bottles that were half full. He also had trouble making sense of the truth behind the façade of my carefully constructed life. The house was tidy, the kids were fed and dressed well, I held down a job and I was looking okay. But my drinking was quite messed up.

Five o'clock—the witching hour I used to call it—that was the magic hour for me when it was okay to have a glass of wine. I got very protective over that time. It was me time, Mummy o'clock, basically. That's when I started to use alcohol to de-stress. It was less about fun and more like *I need this*. I'd think about that first drink of the day all day. It would get me through all those stressful moments. I was all about getting the house ready, cleaned perfectly, dinner perfectly done, a kid perfectly prepared for bed, all so I could have my time.

But then the wheels started coming off. I'd have to cut back on the amount of work that I could do the next day, because I'd need to sleep more. After I got my daughter off to school I'd just crash out for a couple of hours because I literally couldn't function. The last five to ten years of my drinking I was having probably on average about a bottle and a half to sometimes two bottles a night. I'd be pretty knackered the next day—touchy and teary and falling asleep on the couch. But I'd still do it again the next day.

My last night of drinking I had four bottles of wine in one sitting and talked a whole pile of rubbish to Mike, thinking I was being fabulous and clever. He went to bed and I had a strange and eerie sensation of being outside of my body, hovering over and watching myself. I felt nervous and shaky with a foreboding feeling of doom. I was scared. Something in me knew I was going to die unless I stopped drinking. I went to bed, woke with yet another brutal hangover and vowed again that it would be my last one. I was finished. I had had enough of feeling sick and tired and mad. I wanted my life back, whatever that looked like, without alcohol. Mike said he would help and stand by me. It was the first time someone had cared about me enough to hold my hand through the fire of giving it up, and it was his strength and resolve that helped me get back on the road to sobriety.

I saw my doctor straight away and started taking Antabuse [a drug that blocks the effects of alcohol and makes you extremely sick if you drink it]. I believe it saved my life. I sweated through a few sleepless nights and withdrawal symptoms like 'electric fleas', which felt like my skin had been turned inside out. I returned to recovery meetings and started seeing a drug and alcohol counsellor twice a week. Recovery and staying sober was my daily 'job' for about six months. If I wasn't at a meeting, I was reading, watching and listening to recovery material. I needed to fill my head and life up with good, positive stuff to stay on the right track.

I felt awful for the first six months. I was emotionally fragile and battling big time with massive untreated depression and anxiety. I was also perimenopausal and had a lot of pain in my back. I didn't know what was going on for ages, and it's taken me a long time to address all of those things and learn that it can be done without alcohol. I had no idea how to look after myself. I didn't know even basic things like how much sleep to get or how to eat properly, let alone how to be strong, how to grow up, how to trust myself. You can't do those things when you're anaesthetised, which is basically what alcohol does. It took a few years to sort myself out. I had a lot of medical help and wonderful recovery folk helping me to separate my alcoholism from other conditions.

I don't see the people I used to drink with anymore. And new friendships are obviously not based around alcohol; we do different things. It's really refreshing to not have it be all about drink. I really value authentic connection now; I can't be bothered with a lot of fluffing around and fakery. I just feel like I've wasted so much time in my life. Every time I was in trouble, which was all the time, I can trace it back to my use of alcohol. I made dumb decisions. I did stupid things. I let myself down and everyone else down.

I have really strong feelings about alcohol and what it's taken from me. I can see that it takes everything away from you. It rips apart families, takes away self-esteem, takes away health, takes away money, takes away your choices in life. To me it's soul-sucking.

I constantly try to remember to be grateful, and I don't usually have to try. I'm one of those really annoying morning people now, skipping around. I never used to be. I was like something out of *The Walking Dead* in the morning, feeling like crap all the time. Now that I don't feel like that, I'm just so happy. You know, I don't regret for a second giving it away and I never want to touch it again.

39.

No downsides

I was in the middle of writing this book when my social-media accounts lit up. 'Women who give up alcohol have better mental health, study finds'[1] was the first headline I saw, followed swiftly by, 'Quitting alcohol is good for women's health and well-being'.[2] Then, 'Women who completely quit drinking have better mental wellbeing'[3] and 'Giving up alcohol can provide a mental health boost for women'.[4] They kept coming, these articles, thick and fast, as recovery folk across the globe enthusiastically shared the findings of a study published in the *Canadian Medical Association Journal*, everyone so delighted that there was some rock-solid, peer-reviewed, irrefutable, unequivocal research—from a brain scientist no less—proving what we all already knew to be true: that quitting alcohol makes you feel better. Not miserable. Not bereft. Not boring. Not flat. Not like you're missing out. Not like the fun has stopped. None of that. Better, happier, more content, less miserable, healthier, more connected, more well.

Ladies, it's a fact.

I realise there's been quite a lot of gritty talk in this book thus far. Disconnection, vulnerability, assault and trauma—they're not exactly happy-happy-joy-joy topics, are they? Cancer, assault, targeting and manipulation—these are all confronting topics, I get that. But I'm a little bit 'sorry, not sorry' about that. Home truths about alcohol and the impact it's having on our lives need to be said. They need to be shouted from the rooftops, frankly, until they're heard, understood and accepted by everyone, because too many of us are struggling with the way things are now. Too many of us are feeling stuck, miserable and alone. Too many of us are operating below par, often feeling guilty, confused and isolated. All due to that bloody glorified, normalised, readily available, cheap as chips, liquid drug ethanol. Enough already.

So, on the back of a brain scientist's research, and to counteract all the heavy stuff I've been going over in this book so far, I'd like now to inject a bit of positivity. It's time to lighten the mood and end things on an uplifting note. Luckily, that's pretty easy for me to do because I am so happy to have alcohol out of my life! I cannot say it loudly enough: I simply love being sober. And this is really something given how much I used to love my wines.

I love not having to reach for a substance to relax me or lift me up. I love having better strategies for dealing with tough stuff. I love having extra money in my pocket to spend on bath bombs and fancy teas. I love being able to rely on myself at all times to deal with things to the best of my ability. I love not having to check my phone or Facebook account to see if I sent any embarrassing messages the night before. I love kissing my kids goodnight and not breathing wine fumes all over their faces. I love waking up every morning with no hangover. I love knowing myself better and understanding my moods properly for the first time. I love that I get touched by things that are touching, moved by things that are moving, frustrated by things that are frustrating, lifted up by things that are uplifting. I love that I watch TV until late at night and remember what happened. I love that I inwardly flip the bird to every bullshit marketing message trying to catch my eye. I love that I'm part of a cool sober gang of brave and amazing people. I love that it's so cheap when I go out to bars and restaurants now. I love that I'm never slurry or stumbly or embarrassingly sloppy. I love remembering every detail of everything. I love that my skin and hair are healthier and I've lost weight. I love laying my sober head on the pillow at night. I love living sober.

Sometimes people with a glass in their hand ask me if I miss drinking, or they say 'sorry' when pouring a wine in front of me, as if it's hard for me to watch. I try to play it cool, not wanting them to feel bad for drinking (that's their choice and they're entitled to make it), but if only they knew how monumentally happy I am inside to be rid of that stuff. Free from the miserable booze trap I was once in.

There is so much positivity and light that comes from quitting booze. Yes, it's hard work. Yes, it requires a big effort. Yes, we feel raw and vulnerable at first. Yes, we have to go through some awkward social events and extreme emotional times. Yes, things sometimes get worse before they get better. Yes, yes, yes to all of that. But eventually, always eventually, people who have quit drinking start to soar. They emerge happier, healthier, more content and connected to themselves and the people around them. Listen to the brain scientists, listen to the experts, listen to sober people like me who tell you this. There are *no downsides* to quitting booze. None at all. You will get to a place where you don't miss alcohol or hanker for it at all. You will get to a place where you don't envy other people for drinking. You will get to a place where you look at the booze-saturated environment we live in, where alcohol is hailed as this ridiculously great thing, and shake your head in incredulity at a situation that is so harmful and dumb.

Boozing is living a wild, crazy, blurry, knee-jerk, detached and numbed-out life that is sometimes fun and sometimes sad and sometimes downright miserable (when you get to where I was with my habit). Sobriety is not like that. Sobriety is not quick reactions and dramatic developments. Sobriety is all the little things. It's the lovely conversations at the end of a party, the quiet, cosy conversations that are real and memorable. It's getting up at midnight to rub a sick child's back and feeling so grateful to be fully alert. It's delighting in an empty recycling bin. It's driving home at midnight. I love driving home in the dark so much. It's hearing people talk about their own struggles and not inwardly running a mile, but listening, really listening. It's that beautiful moment after you've stared down a craving and resisted the urge to drink, and it's gone away and you realise it was lying to you and you didn't want/need/deserve the drink after all. That is a truly beautiful sober moment. It's waiting—waiting for bad moods to pass, waiting for glum phases to end, waiting for the light to return. Knowing that it always does. It's really appreciating a hot cup of tea, really appreciating each and every sip. Or really appreciating a small sweet square of chocolate as it melts in your mouth. It's looking in the mirror and knowing that whatever is looking back at you is real, not some blurry distant mirage. It's just the underlying beauty of the knowledge that you are sober. You are not drunk anymore; you are sober. That's what sobriety truly is. It's that little gold nugget of truth that you tuck away inside and nurture. *I am not drunk anymore. I am sober.*

A lovely woman called Emma told me recently, 'I wouldn't have the abundance that I have in my life now if I'd carried on drinking. Now I'm in control of any situation. I can feel each moment and understand it. I know I don't have to be happy all the time and I know I don't have to be sad the whole time. I understand my reactions a lot more, and I try to respond, not react. If I work really hard to understand that I've got a part to play, then I can respond so much better. Everyone is going to have stress in their lives, everyone is going to have shit happen. It just keeps on coming. Any excuse to drink will always be there, and we've got to understand that. It's how we deal with life that counts. Yep, it sucks but we can deal with this. Alcohol is only going to drown out any reasonable response.'

If you want to keep on drinking, that is totally your choice. You have a right to make it and please don't feel bad about it. I genuinely mean that. Your life, your choice. But if you have even the slightest bit of sober curiosity, why not give it a try? A decent try—at least six months. Time enough for some moods to come and go, some tricky issues to arise, some celebrations to be had. Time enough that you can move through something normally associated with alcohol, then have time pass so that you can look back in hindsight and reflect.

Finally, it's vital that we women speak openly to one another about alcohol and the impact it's having on our lives. Talk honestly to your girlfriends. Not at 5 p.m. when the chardonnay is flowing and the dopamine is surging. At 9 a.m. after you've slept like crap and your anxiety is peaking. Or at lunchtime during a busy week when your to-do list is crushing you. Be vulnerable and be real. Admit it if you're worried. Admit it if you're struggling. Admit it if you're questioning whether the solution to life's pressure is to be found in a bottle. Cut through the liquid bullshit and really talk.

Ask yourself, is alcohol really delivering everything it promises? Chances are you'll come to realise that the promises of wine o'clock add up to one giant myth.

Acknowledgements

This book is the result of an intense year of work. I spent four months gathering and processing womens' stories, a month or so figuring out how to corral the vast topic of women and alcohol into a logical structure, and eight solid months sitting at my laptop day after day after day, writing.

Thank you to all of the women who have shared their stories, answering my personal questions openly and honestly, and who have allowed their tales to be included even after seeing them laid out in black and white, which I know can be a very confronting thing. Your willingness to open up and be vulnerable will help countless others, and this book would be considerably poorer without your voices.

Thank you to all my other interviewees for adding depth, context and analysis: Steph Anderson, Matt Calman, Professor Jennie Connor, Professor Carol Emslie, Grant Hewison, Dr Nicki Jackson, Sue Kerr, Crystal McLean, Brydie Meinung, Karen Nimmo, Olivia Pennelle, Debora Spar and Jess Stuart.

Thank you to all the other authors, writers, podcasters, researchers, academics and experts who I have quoted. Your work is so important in pushing the truth out.

Thank you to the team at Allen & Unwin for kindly and confidently shepherding me through the whole book-writing process (again)—Jenny Hellen for believing in my idea and encouraging me every step of the way, and Leanne McGregor, Courtney Smith, Erena Shingade and Abba Renshaw.

Thank you to freelance editor Tessa King for your thorough and considered go-through of my manuscript.

Thank you Victoria University of Wellington for unknowingly providing me with the most excellent location in which to research and write. Many hard-working hours were spent on the top floors of your library, looking out over the harbour while pulling thoughts out of my brain.

Thank you to the New Zealand Drug Foundation and Health Promotion Agency for your continued support of Living Sober (livingsober.org.nz). Our community is extremely fortunate to remain free for all because of your backing.

Most of all, thank you to my wonderful husband, Corin Dann. This book would not exist without your love and support. Thank you for listening, advising, reading, commenting, questioning, reassuring and picking up the slack at home while I sweated away at the library. Enjoy your epic Indonesian surf trip—you've earned it!

Find me on Facebook (Mrs D is Going Without), Instagram (@mrs_d_alcoholfree) or Twitter (@mrsdalcoholfree).

Notes

1. Here, there and everywhere

1   Jo Lines-McKenzie, 'One in four hospital ED admissions related to alcohol', Stuff, 20 December 2016, <stuff.co.nz/national/health/87785603/one-in-four-in-hospital-because-of-booze>.

2   Mental Health Foundation of New Zealand, 'Alcohol', last reviewed 28 January 2020, <mentalhealth.org.nz/get-help/a-z/resource/35/alcohol>.

3   Alcohol Healthwatch, 'Our drinking environment', ActionPoint, undated, <actionpoint.org.nz/our-drinking-environment>, citing R. McGee, J. Ketchel and A. I. Reeder, 'Alcohol imagery on New Zealand television', *Substance Abuse Treatment, Prevention, and Policy*, 2007, vol. 2, article 6, <doi.org/10.1186/1747-597X-2-6>.

3. Treat, reward, celebrate, soothe

1   Allen Carr, *The Easy Way to Stop Drinking: A revolutionary new approach to escaping from the alcohol trap*, New York, USA: Sterling Publishing Co. Inc., 2005, p. 69.

2 Annie Grace, *This Naked Mind: Control alcohol, find freedom, discover happiness and change your life*, New York, USA: Penguin Random House, 2018, p. 7.

3 Judith Grisel, *Never Enough: The neuroscience and experience of addiction*, New York, USA: Doubleday, 2019, p. 3.

4 Helidth Ravenholm and Carole Reid, 'Cultural indoctrination—the basic principles', 2016, <www.academia.edu/28179131/cultural_indoctrination_the_basic_principles>.

5. Bonding agent

1 Jacqueline Mroz, *Girl Talk: What science can tell us about female friendship*, Seattle, USA: Seal Press, 2018, p. xiii.

2 Ibid.

3 Megan Peters, 'When book club equals wine club', addiction.com, 20 January 2016, <addiction.com/blogs/expert-blogs/book-club-equals-wine-club>.

4 Emily Nicholls, '"I feel like I have to become part of that identity": Negotiating femininities and friendships through alcohol consumption in Newcastle, UK', *International Journal of Drug Policy*, 19 July 2019, <sciencedirect.com/science/article/abs/pii/S0955395919301975>.

5 Robin McKie, '10,000 years of cheers: Why social drinking is an ancient ritual', *The Guardian*, 1 September 2018, <theguardian.com/society/2018/sep/01/social-drinking-moderation-health-risks>.

7. How did we get here?

1   Ministry for Culture and Heritage, '"Six o'clock swill" begins', last reviewed 25 January 2017, <nzhistory.govt. nz/the-six-oclock-swill-begins>.

2   Brett McEwan, Maxine Campbell, Antonia Lyons and David Swain, *Pleasure, Profit and Pain: Alcohol in New Zealand and the contemporary culture of intoxication*, Hamilton, NZ: University of Waikato Faculty of Arts and Social Sciences, 2013, p. 38.

3   Tom Hunt, 'Alcohol harm more than triple the cost of all Treaty claims so far—economist', Stuff, 17 August 2018, <stuff.co.nz/national/health/106343048/alcohol-harm-more-than-triple-the-cost-of-all-treaty-claims-so-far--economist>.

4   Health Promotion Agency (HPA), 'Key facts about drinking in New Zealand', Alcohol.org.nz, last reviewed 28 January 2020, <alcohol.org.nz/sites/default/files/documents/Key-facts-about-drinking-in-New-Zealand. PDF>.

5   1 *News*, 'Researchers call for Government action on alcohol harm as up to 3000 babies born with alcohol-related brain damage a year', tvnz.co.nz, 27 July 2018, <tvnz.co.nz/one-news/new-zealand/researchers-call-government-action-alcohol-harm-up-3000-babies-born-related-brain-damage-year>.

6   Alcohol Healthwatch, 'Deaths and other harm from alcohol', ActionPoint, undated, <www.actionpoint.org. nz/deaths-from-alcohol>, citing Doug Sellman and Jennie Connor, '*In utero* brain damage from alcohol: A preventable tragedy', *The New Zealand Medical Journal*,

November 2009, vol. 122, no. 1306, <researchgate.net/
publication/41420074_In_utero_brain_damage_from_
alcohol_A_preventable_tragedy>.

7   Health Promotion Agency (HPA), 'Sale and Supply of
    Alcohol Act 2012', Alcohol.org.nz, undated, <alcohol.
    org.nz/management-laws/nz-alcohol-laws/sale-and-
    supply-of-alcohol-act-2012>.

9. It's all about dopamine

1   Judith Grisel, *Never Enough: The neuroscience and experience
    of addiction*, New York, USA: Doubleday, 2019, p. 3.
2   Health Promotion Agency (HPA), *The Straight Up Guide
    to Standard Drinks: Know how much alcohol you're really
    drinking*, April 2016, available at <alcohol.org.nz/help-
    advice/standard-drinks/tool-a-guide-to-standard-
    drinks>.
3   Grisel, *Never Enough*, p. 25.
4   Ibid, p. 28.
5   Susan Peirce Thompson, *Bright Line Eating: The science
    of living happy, thin, and free*, Carlsbad, USA: Hay House
    Inc., 2017, p. 52.
6   Matua Raki, National Addiction Workforce
    Development, *A Guide to the Addiction Treatment Sector in
    Aotearoa New Zealand*, Wellington, New Zealand: Matua
    Raki, 2014, <matuaraki.org.nz/uploads/files/resource-
    assets/a-guide-to-the-addiction-treatment-sector-in-
    aotearoa-new-zealand.pdf>.
7   Drinkaware, 'Alcohol and women', undated,
    <drinkaware.co.uk/alcohol-facts/health-effects-of-
    alcohol/alcohol-and-gender/alcohol-and-women>.

8   Mario Frezza et al., 'High blood alcohol levels in women—the role of decreased gastric alcohol dehydrogenase activity and first-pass metabolism', *The New England Journal of Medicine*, 11 January 1990, vol. 322, no. 2, <nejm.org/doi/full/10.1056/NEJM199001113220205>.

9   J. Milic et al., 'Menopause, ageing, and alcohol use disorders in women', *Maturitas: The European Menopause Journal*, May 2018, vol. 111, <ncbi.nlm.nih.gov/pubmed/29673827>.

10 Daniel W. Hommer, 'Male and female sensitivity to alcohol-induced brain damage', National Institute on Alcohol Abuse and Alcoholism, July 2004, <pubs.niaaa.nih.gov/publications/arh27-2/181-185.htm>.

11 Dr Lars Møller, World Health Organization, 'Q&A—How can I drink alcohol safely?', last reviewed 28 January 2020, <euro.who.int/en/health-topics/disease-prevention/alcohol-use/data-and-statistics/q-and-a-how-can-i-drink-alcohol-safely>.

11. Disconnection

1   Judith Grisel, *Never Enough: The neuroscience and experience of addiction*, New York, USA: Doubleday, 2019, p. 94.

2   Brené Brown, 'The power of vulnerability', TED Talk at TEDxHouston 2010, <ted.com/talks/brene_brown_the_power_of_vulnerability?language=en>.

15. The C words

1   The information in the opening paragraphs of this

chapter has been gleaned from multiple sources: Cancer Research UK, 'Does alcohol cause cancer?', last reviewed 28 December 2018, <cancerresearchuk. org/about-cancer/causes-of-cancer/alcohol-and-cancer/does-alcohol-cause-cancer>; Committee on Carcinogenicity (UK), 'Statement on consumption of alcoholic beverages and risk of cancer', Oxfordshire, UK: Public Health England, 2015, <drugsandalcohol. ie/24998/1/COC_2015_S2__Alcohol_and_Cancer_ statement.pdf>; National Cancer Institute (USA), 'Alcohol and cancer risk', last reviewed 13 September 2018, <cancer.gov/about-cancer/causes-prevention/ risk/alcohol/alcohol-fact-sheet>; Cancer Society (NZ), 'Alcohol and cancer', last reviewed 1 November 2017, <cancernz.org.nz/reducing-cancer-risk/what-you-can-do/alcohol-and-cancer>; Cancer Society (NZ), 'Position statement on alcohol and cancer risk', 6 June 2014, <cancernz.org.nz/assets/Alcohol-and-cancer/Alcohol-and-Cancer-Risk-26Jun2014.pdf>; Breast Cancer Foundation NZ, 'Lower your risk of breast cancer', undated, <breastcancerfoundation.org.nz/breast-awareness/risk-factors/lower-your-risk-of-breast-cancer>.

2   Research New Zealand, *Ready to Contemplate? Midlife adults and their relationship with alcohol*, Wellington, NZ: Health Promotion Agency, 2018, available at <hpa.org. nz/research-library/research-publications/ready-to-contemplate-midlife-adults-and-their-relationship-with-alcohol>.

3   Wikipedia, 'Confirmation bias', last reviewed

17 December 2019, <en.wikipedia.org/wiki/
Confirmation_bias>.

4　Mark Petticrew et al., 'How alcohol industry
organisations mislead the public about alcohol and
cancer', *Drug and Alcohol Review*, March 2018, vol. 37,
no. 3, <onlinelibrary.wiley.com/doi/full/10.1111/
dar.12596>.

5　Ibid.

17. Big Alcohol

1　Christopher Knaus, '"Alcohol industry fingerprints
all over" Australia's plan to tackle overdrinking', *The
Guardian*, 7 August 2019, <theguardian.com/australia-
news/2019/aug/07/alcohol-industry-fingerprints-all-
over-australias-plan-to-tackle-overdrinking>; Rob
Stock, 'Book reveals tobacco industry leagued with
boozemakers to kill New Zealand's Public Health
Commission', Stuff, 17 March 2019, <stuff.co.nz/
business/111290233/book-reveals-tobacco-industry-
leagued-with-boozemakers-to-kill-new-zealands-
public-health-commission>.

2　Farah Hancock, 'Alcohol Act struggles under industry
pressure', Newsroom, last reviewed 12 June 2018,
<newsroom.co.nz/2018/06/10/116707/alcohol-act-
struggles-under-industry-pressure>.

3　For example, the Linden Leaves 'Wellbeing Series' in
partnership with *Good* magazine, Phoenix Organics
and Mission Estate Winery, held in February 2019, see
<good.net.nz/article/linden-leaves-wellbeing-series>.

4　For example, see Lion NZ media release, 'Lifeline

Aotearoa launches world first approach to suicide with "Zero Suicide Workplace"', 1 October 2018, <lionco.com/media-centre/lifeline-aotearoa-launches-world-first-approach-to>.

5   Denis Campbell, 'Alcohol industry "puts pregnant women at risk", researchers say', *The Guardian*, 14 October 2019, <theguardian.com/society/2019/oct/14/alcohol-industry-pregnant-women-research-health>.

6   For example, see The Tomorrow Project, 'Smashed Project launches in NZ', 22 May 2019, <cheers.org.nz/our-work/smashedproject>.

7   For example, see <cheers.org.nz>.

8   For example, see Lion NZ media release, 'Standard drink knowledge lacking in New Zealand', January 2019, <lionco.com/media-centre/standard-drink-knowledge-lacking-in-new-zealand>.

9   For example, see John Anthony, 'Alcohol&Me helping to educate workers about effects of alcohol', Stuff, 13 May 2016, <stuff.co.nz/business/79969670/alchoholme-helping-to-educate-workers-about-effects-of-alcohol>.

10   Sally Casswell and Anna Maxwell, Centre for Social & Health Outcomes Research and Evaluation (SHORE), 'What works to reduce alcohol-related harm and why aren't the policies more popular?', *Social Policy Journal of New Zealand Te Puna Whakaaro*, July 2005, no. 25, <msd.govt.nz/about-msd-and-our-work/publications-resources/journals-and-magazines/social-policy-journal/spj25/what-works-reduce-alcohol-related-harm-25-pages-118-141.html>.

19. Targeting women

1   Brett McEwan, Maxine Campbell, Antonia Lyons and David Swain, *Pleasure, Profit and Pain: Alcohol in New Zealand and the contemporary culture of intoxication*, Hamilton, New Zealand: University of Waikato Faculty of Arts and Social Sciences, 2013, p. 15.

2   Siofra Brennan, '"When everything's an effort, you need Buckfast": Hilarious vintage ads reveal how tonic wines were marketed to bored housewives to make life "much more bearable"', MailOnline, 11 October 2017, <dailymail.co.uk/femail/article-4963470/Vintage-ads-reveal-tonic-wine-housewives-friend.html>.

3   Ann Dowsett Johnston, *Drink: The intimate relationship between women and alcohol*, Sydney, Australia: HarperCollins, 2013, p. 67.

4   Amanda Mare Atkinson et al., *A Rapid Narrative Review of Literature on Gendered Alcohol Marketing and its Effects: Exploring the targeting and representation of women*, London, UK: Institute of Alcohol Studies, October 2019, available online at <ias.org.uk/uploads/pdf/IAS%20 reports/rp39102019.pdf>.

5   Irina Gonzalez, 'Ten gross examples of gendered alcohol marketing', The Temper, last reviewed on 28 January 2020, <thetemper.com/10-gross-examples-of-gendered-alcohol-marketing/>.

6   Katie Warren, 'Millennials are spending less money on alcohol than previous generations. Now, brands are marketing their booze as "wellness" drinks in a desperate bid to capture the market', *Business Insider Australia*, 3 June 2019, <businessinsider.com.au/

brands-marketing-alcohol-wellness-drinks-appeal-to-millennials-2019-5>.

7   Cristina Lombardo, 'Gender preferences in wine marketing', paper presented to the Faculty of the Agribusiness Department, California Polytechnic State University (in partial fulfillment of the requirements for the Bachelor of Science), June 2012 <pdfs.semanticscholar.org/85b9/4cfbc70b6e10c659a79f48d877974bddb11a.pdf>.

8   The videos are available at Diageo, 'Celebrating International Women's Day 2019: #BalanceforBetter', 4 March 2019, <diageo.com/en/news-and-media/features/celebrating-international-women-s-day-2019-balanceforbetter/>.

9   'How alcohol companies are using International Women's Day to sell more drinks to women', The Conversation, 8 March 2019, <theconversation.com/how-alcohol-companies-are-using-international-womens-day-to-sell-more-drinks-to-women-113081>.

10 For example, see Newsbeat, 'BrewDog's mock Pink IPA "beer for girls" splits opinion', BBC News, 6 March 2018, <bbc.com/news/newsbeat-43300969>.

21. Warrior Mums of the world, unite

1   'Dear Metro: "How am I supposed to hang out with my 'wine mum' friends now I'm sober?"', Metro, 18 September 2019 <metromag.co.nz/society/society-society/dear-metro-wine-mum-drinking-alcohol-sober-sobriety>.

2   Halley Bondy, 'Wine mom culture is terrible but moms' quiet suffering is worse', The Temper, 9 September 2019, <thetemper.com/wine-mom-culture-quiet-suffering>.

23. #dontpinkmydrink

1   Nicholas Carah et al., 'Emerging social media "platform" approaches to alcohol marketing: A comparative analysis of the activity of the top 20 Australian alcohol brands on Facebook (2012–2014)', *Critical Public Health*, 2018, vol. 28, no. 1, <tandfonline.com/doi/full/10.1080/0 9581596.2017.1282154>.

2   Pew Research Center, 'Social media fact sheet', 12 June 2019, <pewinternet.org/fact-sheet/social-media>.

3   Toby Cox, 'How social media can help businesses win loyal customers', The Manifest, 7 August 2019, <themanifest.com/social-media/how-social-media-can-help-businesses-win-loyal-customers>.

25. Liquid courage

1   Catharine Fairbairn and Michael Sayette, 'A social-attributional analysis of alcohol response', *Psychological Bulletin*, September 2014, vol. 140, no. 5, <researchgate. net/publication/265256946_A_Social-Attributional_ Analysis_of_Alcohol_Response>.

27. The Superwoman problem

1   Debora Spar, quoted in 'The Superwoman myth', Big Think, 6 January 2014, last reviewed 28 January, <bigthink.com/specific-gravity/the-superwoman-myth>.

2   Ibid.

29. Self-medicating

1   Olivia Pennelle, 'When getting sober reveals an underlying illness', The Fix, 9 May 2019, last reviewed 28 January 2020, <thefix.com/when-getting-sober-reveals-underlying-illness>.

2   Matua Raki, National Addiction Workforce Development, 'Co-existing mental health, substance use and gambling problems are the rule not the exception', Matua Raki, undated, <matuaraki.org.nz/uploads/files/resource-assets/co-existing-problems-poster-A3.pdf>.

3   Janice Withnall, 'Preventing more midlife women suffering alcohol-related brain damage through earlier treatment for anxiety and alcohol misuse', 2015, article provided to the author.

31. Adverse Childhood Experiences

1   Vincent J. Felitti et al., 'Relationship of childhood abuse and household dysfunction to many of the leading causes of death in adults', American Journal of Preventive Medicine, May 1998, vol. 14, no. 4, <ajpmonline.org/article/S0749-3797(98)00017-8/fulltext>.

2   M. C. Walsh et al., Adverse Childhood Experiences and School Readiness Outcomes: Results from the Growing Up in New Zealand study, Wellington, NZ: Ministry of Social Development, April 2019, <msd.govt.nz/documents/about-msd-and-our-work/publications-resources/research/children-and-families-research-fund/children-and-families-research-fund-report-adverse-childhood-experiences-and-school-readiness-outcomes-april-2019-final.pdf>.

3   Nadine Burke Harris, 'How childhood trauma affects health across a lifetime', TED Talk at TEDMED 2014, <ted.com/talks/nadine_burke_harris_how_childhood_trauma_affects_health_across_a_lifetime>.

4   Vincent J. Felitti, *The Origins of Addiction: Evidence from the Adverse Childhood Experiences Study*, California, USA: Department of Preventive Medicine, 16 February 2004, <harmreductiontherapy.org/wp-content/uploads/2014/11/Origins-of-Addiction-ACE-Study.pdf>, p. 11.

5   Olivia Pennelle, *Breaking free: Your recovery. Your way* podcast, <stitcher.com/podcast/anchor-podcasts/breaking-free-your-recovery-your-way/e/65057941>; <stitcher.com/podcast/anchor-podcasts/breaking-free-your-recovery-your-way/e/64434757>.

6   Brené Brown, *Braving the Wilderness: The quest for true belonging and the courage to stand alone*, London, UK: Vermilion, 2017, pp. 66–67.

33. The ultimate rebellion

1   Sarah Hepola, *Blackout: Remembering the things I drank to forget*, London, UK: Two Roads Books, 2015, p. 217.

39. No downsides

1   Adam Forrest, 'Women who give up alcohol have better mental health, study finds', *The Independent*, 8 July 2019, <independent.co.uk/news/health/alcohol-women-give-up-drinking-mental-health-abstinence-study-a8992561.html>.

2   'Quitting alcohol is good for women's health and well-being, study says', IFL Science!, 8 July 2019, < iflscience.

com/health-and-medicine/quitting-alcohol-is-good-for-womens-health-and-wellbeing-study-says>.

3   Natasha Hinde, 'Women who completely quit drinking have better mental wellbeing, study suggests', HuffPost, last reviewed 9 July 2019, <huffingtonpost. co.uk/entry/women-who-completely-quit-drinking-have-better-mental-wellbeing-study-suggests_ uk_5d22ff62e4b04c481416a591>.

4   'Giving up alcohol can provide a mental health boost for women', France Surgery, 11 July 2019, <france-surgery.com/en/news-giving-up-alcohol-can-provide-a-mental-health-boost-for-women-791.php>.

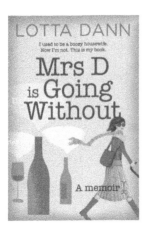

An honest, upfront, engaging account of a
suburban housewife's journey from miserable
wine-soaked boozer to self-respecting sober lady.

Lotta Dann was in trouble—her fun drinking habit had slowly morphed into an obsessive hunger for wine. One bottle a night was never quite enough. When she tried to cut down, she found it nearly impossible to have an alcohol-free day.

Everyone around could see her drinking, but no one realised what a serious problem it was. She was high-functioning, fun-loving Lotta, not some messy, hopeless drunk. Only Lotta knew how sick and twisted her thinking about wine had become.

Desperate and miserable, she was falling deeper and deeper into a boozy hellhole and running out of ideas about what she could do to stop it. What's a girl to do when her beloved wine becomes the enemy?

Here's what Lotta did. She stopped drinking and secretly started a blog that charted the highs and lows of learning to live without alcohol. Mrs D was anonymous, honest and, as Lotta would discover, surrounded by people who would help her on her journey, and whom she could help in return.

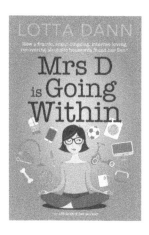

Lotta Dann should have it all sorted. She's quit a dysfunctional drinking habit, has written a bestselling memoir and has launched a website to help others get sober. Life should be sweet, right? Wrong.

Despite outward appearances, three years after getting sober Lotta is struggling to deal with life in the raw. It's becoming abundantly clear what people mean when they say that putting down the drink is just the beginning.

Truth is, Lotta's lifelong heavy-drinking habit has left her as a fledgling emotionally. She's slowly accepting that she needs to do some more work on herself. But what? Please don't say it has to involve turning into a hippy. Can't she just comfort herself with another chocolate muffin, distract herself on Instagram and hope for the best? It would appear not.

In *Mrs D Is Going Within* Lotta outlines the practices she developed and strategies she worked on to start establishing herself as an emotionally robust woman.

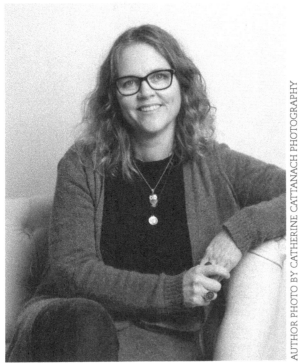

Lotta Dann has a degree in broadcasting and communications and a master's degree in film, television and media studies. She worked as a TV journalist, producer and director until she got sober aged 39, at which point her career changed as much as her interior life did. She now works largely from her home in the hills of Wellington, New Zealand, which she shares with her husband, three sons and a black Labrador. She runs busy social-media accounts promoting recovery, manages the highly successful online community Living Sober (livingsober.org.nz), and lately has been taking regular trips away to run day-long workshops on addiction and recovery. This is her third book.